The Cancer Journey

The Cancer Journey

Understanding Diagnosis, Treatment, Recovery, and Prevention

Chadi Nabhan, MD, MBA, FACP

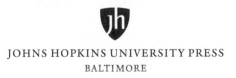

JOHNS HOPKINS UNIVERSITY PRESS
BALTIMORE

Note to the Reader: This book is not meant as a substitute for medical care or as an alternative to official medical advice from your physician. No treatment, diagnostic test, decision, or follow-up should be based solely on this book. Instead, this book can be used as a resource that might help you as you receive the formal recommendations from your medical care team. It is written as a companion to help you navigate the medical journey when you or your loved ones are faced with cancer.

The author and publisher have made reasonable efforts to determine that the drugs discussed in the book conform to the practices of the general oncology community. Some drugs that are mentioned may not be officially approved by the Food and Drug Administration for the indication discussed. Some information might be outdated by the time you read this book as scientific advances progress rapidly, and consulting your doctor about all the information you consume in this book is critical for optimal utilization. To gain more information about any drug mentioned in the book, I urge you to check the package insert and read all necessary details.

© 2024 Johns Hopkins University Press
All rights reserved. Published 2024
Printed in the United States of America on acid-free paper
9   8   7   6   5   4   3   2   1

Johns Hopkins University Press
2715 North Charles Street
Baltimore, Maryland 21218
www.press.jhu.edu

Library of Congress Cataloging-in-Publication Data

Names: Nabhan, Chadi, author.
Title: The cancer journey : understanding diagnosis, treatment, recovery, and
    prevention / Chadi Nabhan.
Description: Baltimore : Johns Hopkins University Press, 2024. |
    Series: A Johns Hopkins Press health book | Includes bibliographical
    references and index.
Identifiers: LCCN 2024001338 | ISBN 9781421449753 (hardcover) |
    ISBN 9781421449760 (paperback) | ISBN 9781421449777 (ebook)
Subjects: LCSH: Cancer—Popular works.
Classification: LCC RC263 .N33 2024 | DDC 616.99/4—dc23/eng/20240301
LC record available at https://lccn.loc.gov/2024001338

A catalog record for this book is available from the British Library.

Special discounts are available for bulk purchases of this book.
For more information, please contact Special Sales at specialsales@jh.edu.

To my parents, who brought me into this world and made
me the man that I am. You guided me and continue
to do so. I yearn to see your happiness and smiles
and strive to rise to your expectations.

To my family, my wife, and my kids, who supported me
and loved me through the ups, the downs, and the
turns. I hope to return the favor one day.

To my friends and loved ones, who believed in me,
tolerated me, and never doubted me.

To my patients, who taught me, inspired me,
trusted me, and made me a better human.

I owe you and I love you all.

Contents

Preface

There are many great books written about cancer. You may ask, "What is so special about this one?"

Simply put, I share over 20 years of experience as a cancer doctor in a simplified and easy-to-read format. Through storytelling of real-life clinical scenarios, I take the reader through the journey of a cancer diagnosis, from A to Z.

My goal is to bring the reader into the exam room to experience what actually happens at the point the unfortunate diagnosis is shared, how oncologists use information that affects clinical decision-making, and how the human element of medicine and oncology is part of this journey. In doing so, my hope is to simplify a very complex and emotional situation so that patients and families are better prepared to understand and question the diagnosis, the treatment, and other aspects of cancer care.

I start by explaining what cancer is. What is that disease that poses an immediate scare in us once we hear the "c" word? Why does it develop; can we prevent it; and what can we do as far as screening in healthy people? What are the symptoms and signs of cancer; how do we make a diagnosis; what should you expect during your first oncology visit, and what questions should you ask; how do doctors stage cancer; what about second opinions and clinical trials; and how do we decide on treatment? Once we decide to treat, what about chemotherapy, radiation, surgery, immunotherapy, hormonal therapy, targeted therapy, cellular therapy, and bone marrow transplantation? Readers should become familiar with all these concepts, delivered in a digestible and uncomplicated manner. This information should arm everyone interested with the knowledge needed as they navigate this unexpected journey.

I also discuss alternative and complementary therapies. These are top of mind for any patient diagnosed with cancer, but there is so much noise that can add to the bewilderment. I do my best to minimize the confusion. What is the role of yoga, massage therapy, pet therapy, acupuncture, and vitamins? Does sugar cause cancer? I have heard these and other questions from my patients, families, and even healthcare providers.

I devote an entire chapter to communication and another to survivorship. Optimizing how we communicate with patients is critical, as the journey has its ups and downs, and explaining these nuances can be challenging and emotionally charged. I share my own stories where patients felt that I had failed to communicate. Every story was a lesson that helped me do better with the next patient. I kept two folders in my desk drawer: one with greeting cards and thank-you notes from patients, and the other with personal notes from patients and families who thought I had failed them. I read the second folder often to stay grounded and to remind myself that I could always do better. Based on my experience and published evidence, I propose various ways to improve the sacred relationship between the oncologist and their patients.

It is never easy to talk about palliative and hospice care, but it is essential to address the elephant in the room when all treatments fail and our focus shifts to helping patients manage the symptoms while recognizing that the cancer has won. I describe these challenges and suggest that there is always a silver lining, even in the darkest of moments.

The last chapter is about future directions in cancer care. It is not easy to forecast the future, but I attempt to bring my own clinical expertise, research work, and knowledge of the field, and propose several areas where our cancer care might shift and change. I am certain

I was not inclusive of every possibility, but I did my best to capture the essence of our scientific and care delivery progress.

At the end of each chapter, I provide a brief summary of "take-home points" that helps to capture the essence of the chapter. There are references for each chapter for those who want to take a deeper dive into a particular topic, but the goal is to ensure simplicity in explaining the science and for the book to be a resource to everyone affected or interested in cancer and advances in its treatment.

None of us wants to get sick—and if we do, none of us wants to get cancer. Let's face it, no matter how much we try explaining, that diagnosis will change your life and the lives of your loved ones forever. If this book makes the journey easier, less stressful, more palatable, and better to navigate, then it was well worth the two years it took me to write these words.

Whether you are a patient, a family member, a student, a nurse, a pharmacist, a doctor, or any healthcare professional, I hope you find some knowledge and solace between these pages, and I hope that you finish the book knowing more than when you started reading. I hope that you will witness how much progress has been made in science and oncology.

Introduction

"IF THERE IS A DOCTOR on the plane, please press the button for the flight attendant," announced the pilot on my flight back to Chicago from an international scientific conference I was attending.

As an oncologist, I've always felt that I can't contribute much to medical emergencies; I am not a cardiologist or an intensivist and have not stayed up to date with the latest scientific advances on how to handle life-threatening emergencies. But the guilt of not responding always got the best of me. The pilot did not specify a specialty, and I am a doctor, after all. I pressed the button hesitantly, hoping that other specialists on this large trans-Atlantic flight might have done the same. Looks like I was the only doctor on this plane. Not cool.

Within seconds, a United flight attendant appeared in front of me and took me to the first-class cabin, where I saw an ill-appearing, pale, weak, and dizzy passenger. I was pleasantly surprised when the flight attendant gave me a stethoscope and a blood pressure machine that were stored on board. There were also some standard medications like aspirin, acetaminophen, blood pressure pills, and other medications to treat urgent symptoms. After taking a brief history of the man, I could tell that he was severely dehydrated and needed fluids. He had suffered bad bouts of diarrhea all night long after a questionable meal. The flight attendant informed me that they had saline on the plane, and because it had been more than a decade since I had last started an IV line on a patient, I embarrassingly inquired if a nurse was flying with us; the odds were good since we had over 300 passengers returning to O'Hare. Nurses have always been better than me at starting IV lines, and many have taught me, among other things, how to do so. It was my lucky day. One intensive care unit (ICU) nurse was on board, and another retired trauma nurse was also returning from Europe. The patient got his saline, and his blood pressure started to improve. I returned to my seat, feeling triumphant and satisfied.

I had managed not to talk with my fellow passenger for the first six hours of the flight, but this incident sparked his interest. I had the aisle seat, and he had been resting in the middle, with his wife to his right snoozing on and off by the window. As I settled back in my seat, he turned toward me and asked, "So, what specialty are you in? My son wants to go to medical school."

"I am an oncologist," I responded.

"Wow, that's great. Where do you practice?"

"I am at the University of Chicago." It was 2015, and I was a faculty member there focusing on lymphomas. I was returning from the International Congress on Malignant Lymphoma, which is held bi-annually in the beautiful town of Lugano, Switzerland. I was lucky to have attended that conference since 2005 and fortunate to occasionally present some of my research findings there.

At this, his wife perked up and started listening; she was no longer sleepy.

After telling me about his son's aspirations and me sharing a few pointers on what to do and what not to do when pursuing this career, he gave me a puzzled look and shot a question, as if demanding an immediate answer: "Why can't you guys cure cancer with all this research you do?"

I heard his wife whisper to him, "Can we please stop talking about the 'c' word and leave the doctor alone?"

He shrugged and asked her to stay quiet, looking at me with anticipation.

"But we do cure many cancers; we actually do. We don't cure all, but we cure some." I said, defending my profession and specialty.

"I lost so many relatives to cancer. Maybe it runs in my family." He shook his head, unconvinced by my defense.

"See, not all cancers are the same," I said. "It is kind of an unfair question. Every cancer is different, and every cancer can be cured; it is just that the percentage of cure varies between cancers and between people. There are no easy answers to your question," I continued, "but there are many cancers today that can be handled as chronic diseases, and patients can live long, fruitful lives despite the cancer. So many new treatments exist; the advances are unprecedented."

He shook his head skeptically again as he appeared ready to nap again. "I hope you're right. I am not sure what my son wants to do, but I hope he gets into medical school first. Cancer is a death sentence if you ask me," he mumbled.

It is not an uncommon question for the lay public to ask as to why we have not cured cancer. There is some sense that cancer is one disease, just like a heart attack or asthma. Like my fellow passenger, some people think a cancer diagnosis is the end of life. The reality is different, but this encounter got me thinking about how best to simplify explaining cancer—a disease that takes the lives of many patients every year—to the masses.

I checked back on my first-class patient, who seemed to be doing better. He asked for my card, and I gave it to him, wondering if he would ever call. Maybe he will donate to my research fund, I thought. He never called or donated, but I did get a thank-you letter from United stating they had added 5,000 miles to my mileage plus account.

Back home, I returned to my routine of doing research and administrative work and seeing patients and their families to make diagnoses and recommend treatments. Often, I would get similar questions to the one my fellow flight passenger asked me. These questions conveyed a sense of confusion and uncertainty, but there was never enough time to explain all the important nuances and details of all cancers and their treatments in a way that becomes a guide to the common person.

Until now.

I decided to embark on the journey of writing a guide to cancer basics, from A to Z. But don't worry—this is not a textbook, nor will you be tested on any of the chapters. There won't be any complicated figures or graphs that will make you scratch your head and wonder what you have just read.

My goal is to simplify a complex disease and entity. Cancer, like many other ailments, changes our life trajectory. It is a journey filled with bumps but also with victories. There are many myths about this disease that inflicts almost 2 million Americans every year. And I am here to make the journey smoother, easier, more informative, and free of myths and biases.

Why now? Because the advances in cancer diagnostics and therapeutics are extraordinary, and I am not exaggerating. With that, complexity increases, and it can be more challenging for patients and families to decipher the details and understand all the relevant aspects. Some might not even feel comfortable asking all their questions, or don't know what questions to ask. We cure and control more cancers than we have ever been able to, and my hope is that we continue to do so. I also had the opportunity in recent years to serve as an expert witness in trials where patients sued Monsanto alleging that Roundup, the common weedkiller, caused their lymphoma (see my book *Toxic Exposure* [Johns Hopkins University Press, 2023]). In all these trials, I had to explain basics of cancer development and its therapies to a jury of laypeople. The simplicity of explaining a complex topic was key to conveying important information to the jury.

That experience solidified to me the importance of simple explanations and how far they can go when talking to nonmedical audiences. People want to know and understand, but it's how you deliver the information and explain the facts that matters. For all these reasons, it's time for a book for the people who need it most. For the patients and their loved ones. For primary care doctors who need to explain a complex disease to a long-term patient they cared for before a cancer diagnosis. For anyone who wants simplified answers to complex cancer-related questions.

I am a board-certified internist, hematologist, and medical oncologist. I practiced oncology for almost two decades in a variety of settings: community practice and academic institutions. I conducted research and taught medical students, residents, and fellows in training. I had increased administrative responsibilities even after I had left the university setting and worked in other healthcare sectors. I understand the complexity of the healthcare ecosystem because I worked in all these venues. Throughout my career, my goal was to make a difference in patients' care and lives; to be a valuable resource to patients and their families. If I had helped one patient, one family along the way, then it was well worth the ride.

My own family has been affected by cancer, so I am fully aware of what you might be going through, whether you're a patient or a family member. I wrote this book so that it will be by your side as you embark on this unexpected journey. I want to make an unfortunate event a less unfortunate one. My hope is that this book answers some questions you may have and is there for you every step of the way.

I start by simplifying cancer as a disease and try to explain what cancer is. I then move on to exploring the journey that starts by screening for cancer, developing symptoms, getting tested, receiving the proper diagnosis, and undergoing staging before the needed treatment—surgery, chemotherapy, radiation, or a combination of the three—is initiated. I simplify how we conduct clinical trials and address the importance of second opinions. I also examine the need to monitor for possible recurrence and tackle the problems that patients who survive cancer face. What happens when the journey is complete and there are no more treatments and no more monitoring?

I have always said that we are all either current patients, future patients, or past patients. This book is dedicated to all of us, the patients of yesterday, today, and tomorrow.

CHAPTER 1

What Is Cancer and What Causes It?

The only true wisdom is in
knowing you know nothing.

—*Socrates*

ONE DAY, I GOOGLED "what is cancer?" and within 0.86 seconds, I got back 877 million results. While most patients likely type in the search engine the specific cancer they are suffering from, some might research the general topic when faced with this illness; I wanted to see and read the information they consume. There was clearly no shortage of internet sources trying to explain the word "cancer," and yet I was witnessing much confusion in my clinic when this term was thrown around by patients and their families.

Every organ in our body is composed of cells. Think of the organ as a building and of the cells as the bricks that form the shape of the building. These cells generally live in harmony whereby there is a balance between cell survival and cell death. Cells in each organ have a natural life cycle, and when they die they are replaced by newly formed cells, like the bricks that might have a normal life span before wear and tear requires them to be replaced by new bricks. This distinctive balance is what makes the human body a unique and fascinating machinery. But at times this balance is tipped the wrong way, and the cells continue to grow without their natural death. As these cells continue to multiply, growths are formed, and we call these *tumors*.

Some of these tumors are benign. Benign tumors don't cause much damage, don't spread to other organs, and have little to no impact on a person's life or health. They may be bothersome aesthetically or cause some discomfort based on their location, but they do not threaten someone's life, unless they grow in a vital organ where they may cause a threat (think of the heart as an example). Other tumors are malignant or cancerous, in that they cause health damage, can spread to different organs, and pose a serious threat to someone's health.

Because our body is composed of cells, cancer can develop in any organ. It can start almost anywhere—in the eyes, nose, ovaries, prostate, colon, bones, skin, and so on. No organ is immune from its cells potentially becoming cancerous. These cancer cells that originate in one organ can travel throughout the bloodstream or lymph channels to other organs and metastasize. Sometimes cancer cells travel only to nearby organs and/or lymph nodes close to their origin, but other times they can travel to farther locations in the body.

I realized the importance of explaining that nuance early on in my training, when I was seeing a patient with lung cancer that had gone to the bones. He was accompanied by his wife and two sons. "What are we going to do about my bone cancer?" he asked.

CN: You don't have bone cancer. You have lung cancer that has spread to the bones.

Patient: But the cancer has gone to the bone; does this mean that I don't have bone cancer?

CN: I know what you're saying, but it is still lung cancer that has gone to the bones. You don't have bone cancer. We will need to treat your condition like we treat lung cancers, although there may be some specific therapies that help stop its spread to the remaining healthy bones, and we could administer those too.

I still sensed some confusion and explained further to ensure that he and his family understood that we treated the cancer based on where the tumor had originated. "Many cancers, such as prostate, breast, and thyroid, can spread to the bones. We treat these cancers differently because they originate from different organs," I continued.

Some of this, to some extent, has changed in recent years, where occasionally we treat cancers based on the mutations that led to their development regardless of which organ the cancer had originated from. In other words, we treat these cancers not based on their location but based on what led the cancerous cells to grow uncontrollably. I will explain this concept in future chapters, especially as it has gained momentum in recent years.

So, How Does Cancer Develop?

What makes a normal cell grow uncontrollably is not always known and continues to be the subject of constant research. If you think about it, cancer develops either because the cells do not die like they should or because they continue to grow. Sometimes it is a combination of both.

Largely, cancer occurs because of some damage to the cells whereby they start growing fast and do not continue through their normal life cycle. There is something called programmed cell death, where cells are programmed to die naturally (scientifically, the process is called *apoptosis*) but something happens, and the programmed plan becomes dysfunctional. This occurs because the genes that control cell growth and death are damaged or affected abnormally, so they don't function properly. Some genes normally protect cells from this uncontrollable growth; they act like brake pedals (scientists call them *tumor suppressors*). But when these genes are damaged, they cannot offer such protection. Other genes, when activated, can lead to cell growth and multiplication (scientists call these *oncogenes*).

Genes are arranged one after another on structures inside the cells, called *chromosomes*. An international research effort called the Human Genome Project, which worked to identify the genes contained in the human body, estimated that humans have between 20,000 and 25,000 genes. Each cell normally contains 23 pairs of chromosomes. Twenty-two of these pairs look the same in both males and females. The twenty-third pair, called the sex chromosomes, differs between males and females. Females have two copies of what we call the X chromosome, while males have one X and one Y chromosome.

Genes are composed of DNA. These genes get passed from parents to children and lead to specific traits in the offspring. The critical information that DNA carries is stored as a code composed of four chemical unit bases. Human DNA consists of about 3 billion bases, and more than 99% of those bases are the same in all people. How these bases are placed and their order is oftentimes important for life and death.

The information contained within a gene is essential for genes to produce molecules called *proteins*. Two steps lead to producing proteins: transcription and translation. These two steps combined are known as *gene expression*. During transcription, the information is passed on from the DNA to another molecule called RNA (which is composed of unit bases as well, but slightly different from those of DNA). Think of the RNA as the messenger that contains the information sent from the DNA so that proteins can be formed.

This messenger RNA interacts with other molecules in the cell, eventually leading to the assembly of the protein; this is the translation step.

Proteins are complex molecules that play a critical role in the body; they are made up of hundreds or thousands of amino acids. There are 20 types of amino acids, and their combinations make the protein. The sequence of these amino acids determines each protein. What happens to these proteins can determine which cancer develops and how it will behave. An easier way to think about this is that a gene is a packet of information coding generally for a protein. The protein that's produced is supposed to carry out a specific function. Sometimes, one gene can produce multiple proteins. Of course, there are genes that don't even make proteins. They make RNAs that have some other functional role.

Cancer cells can grow on their own and can trick the immune system, which normally fights foreign invaders, to throw our bodies off balance. In fact, this is exactly why so much research has been dedicated to fighting cancer by stimulating the immune system and priming it to do the job that it was supposed to do. Also, as we age, the ability of our cells to fight what disrupts how they are regulated could deteriorate. Like the bricks on a building, as they age they become damaged. Therefore, we see cancer more often in older people. Each person's cancer has a unique combination of genetic changes. As the cancer continues to grow, additional changes will occur. Even within the same tumor, different cells may have different genetic changes.

To summarize, our cells should live in harmony with adequate balance. When the balance is off, however, cells can continue to multiply uncontrollably or refuse to die naturally. Continued DNA damage leads to the development of cancers. We refer to this damage in the DNA code as mutations. Some would also label these mutations as "driver mutations" if we are certain they are behind the development and progression of a specific cancer. Scientists believe that some of these mutations in the DNA cause no harm and resolve on their own; in other words: our bodies detect these mutations and repair them, so no harm is done. It becomes critical to know whether a mutation is indeed causing a cancer or simply is a bystander. Mutated DNA leads to proteins that are not doing their job properly. Proteins that are not properly functioning can contribute to cancer evolution.

But why do these genes start acting in a weird way, making the cells behave unnaturally? Most often, we don't know, but that does not mean we cannot theorize. Sometimes harmful substances that we are exposed to throughout life can damage the cells. Examples are tobacco, some chemical exposures, pesticides, and even the sun, which damages the skin and can lead to various skin cancers. Sometimes viruses or bacteria contribute to developing cancers. In fact, one of the non-Hodgkin lymphomas (a cancer of the bone marrow and the lymph glands) called MALToma, which affects mainly the stomach lining, is caused by the same bacteria that causes ulcers, namely *Helicobacter pylori*. The first treatment offered to patients suffering from this disease is antibiotics to eradicate this bacterium, and they indeed work in most cases.

When I was a fellow at Northwestern University in the late 1990s, I took care of many patients who developed cancers because their immune system was damaged by HIV. You could argue that some of these cancers never would have developed had it not been for HIV. We can safely assume that conditions that suppress the immune system (some medications do that) could increase the risk of developing some cancers.

I would argue that the most commonly asked question by any patient I have encountered was, "Doc, why did I get this cancer?" This question is often magnified when the affected person is young, lived a healthy lifestyle, exercised regularly, and had no family history. Sadly, the most common answer is, "I don't really know."

I was an attending physician at Advocate Health Care. It was a bit after midnight when my pager angrily beeped. It was the ER physician telling me about a 24-year-old patient who was brought in because of high fevers, fatigue, and headaches. Laboratory studies showed very high white blood cell counts.

"I am coming in," I told the ER doctor.

"Why?" he asked. "We can take care of things until the morning."

"He might have leukemia, and I am concerned about the symptoms you're describing," I said. "I need to see him, examine him, look at his blood, and do a bone marrow biopsy in the morning."

It was morning already, though the sun was not up yet.

I soon diagnosed the patient with an acute form of leukemia; he was young, healthy, an athlete, with no medical issues or a hint of cancer in his family. I am always humbled by how little we know despite how much we think we know. I bring up this story because it is very common for healthy people with no family history to be surprised when diagnosed with cancer. People assume that living healthy is sufficient, but unfortunately, this is not the case. When we take care of ourselves, exercise, eat healthy, and avoid harmful habits, all of this helps, but it never eliminates the possibility of developing cancer.

Nonetheless, there are some risk factors for developing various cancers; I would argue that some risk factors are causative while others are not. Let me elaborate.

Age, for example, is a risk factor for developing cancer, but this does not mean that age by itself causes the cancer. We can argue that an older person had lived long enough to be exposed to many environmental factors that might cause cancer, or that age may have led to some of the genetic machinery to start acting strangely, but I don't think we can look a patient in the eye and tell them that they got cancer simply because they were old. A mutation must have occurred that led to the development of the cancer. Whether said mutation occurred simply because of age and the body's inability to fight it or repair it, or because of some other factors, cannot be answered broadly, but it can only be determined on a case-by-case basis.

In my view, the best way to look at risk factors for cancers is to divide them into causative and non-causative. In other words, some risk factors can cause the cancer, while others are associated with the cancer because of its prevalence in a specific age group, race, or gender.

Then, there are causative risk factors such as the virus and bacteria examples I provided. Additionally, sun exposure can cause skin cancers, and smoking can cause some forms of lung and bladder cancers, among others. Few studies have linked obesity to some cancers, but not all. It is usually impossible to know exactly why one person develops cancer and another does not. We would love to be able to answer all questions, but we can't.

It's unreasonable to list all potential causes for all cancers, since we don't know causations for many and since what causes one cancer might not cause another, and what causes it in one person may not cause it in another. Here are the most common ones talked about and the ones that patients and their families inquire about the most:

- **Tobacco**: Let's not fool ourselves; there is no safe tobacco product. People should avoid all tobacco products. Tobacco-related illnesses are the leading preventable cause of death in the United States, accounting for about 1 in 5 deaths each year. According to the American Cancer Society, tobacco causes about 20% of all cancers and about 30% of all cancer deaths in the

United States. Not all cancers of course are associated with smoking, but many are. Most notable is lung cancer, 80% of which is caused by smoking.

- **Alcohol**: Alcohol is responsible for 6% of all cancer incidence and 4% of all cancer deaths in the United States. Many cancers are not linked to excessive alcohol use, but some are. Studies have shown that the amount of alcohol someone drinks over time, not the type of alcoholic beverage, seems to be the most important factor in raising cancer risk. How alcohol increases the risk of developing some cancers is not well known.

- **Obesity**: Some cancers are linked to obesity. Maintaining a healthy lifestyle, proper diet, and exercise should help reduce many diseases, including some cancers. In research studies, investigators measure obesity using a formula called body mass index (BMI), which is a calculation that incorporates someone's weight and height to reach a number. If that number is 30 or over, the individual is labeled as obese. As I have stated, studies have never consistently determined whether obesity indeed causes cancer, largely because every person's weight fluctuates with time, and it becomes difficult to deduce the impact of obesity on cancer evolution. It is fair to say that there is more evidence that obesity plays a role in some cancers (gallbladder, for example) than in others (leukemia and lymphoma, for example).

- **Sun exposure and ultraviolet (UV) light**: Sun and UV light can cause cancers, mainly skin cancers. I recognize how nice it would be to lie in the sun on the beach, and maybe every so often you need to do so, but sunbathing regularly is damaging to the skin and can lead to various skin cancers. Under no circumstances are tanning beds ever recommended.

- **Cancers from prior cancer therapies**: We use chemotherapies and other modalities to treat cancers, but these treatments can lead to different types of cancers down the road. Therefore, patients with cancers need lifelong monitoring for any potential lasting effects from prior therapies. In fact, this is part of the survivorship programs that I discuss in a future chapter.

- **Viruses**: Viruses such as HIV and human papillomavirus (HPV), among others, have been associated with increased risk of some cancers.

- **Bacteria**: As I mentioned, the bacteria *H. pylori* has been associated with various forms of stomach cancers. There is significant research attempting to understand the association between various pathogens and the development of cancers.

- **Family history**: A family history of cancer might increase the risk of developing that cancer in the patient's relatives. This is different from hereditary causes, and it can be related to family members being exposed to similar environmental factors, although this association is not confirmed.

- **Environmental factors**: Environmental causes can include pesticides and herbicides. For example, the herbicide Roundup has been linked to non-Hodgkin lymphoma.

The simplest way to explain cancer is that it is a disease that could develop in any of our organs due to uncontrollable cell growth or lack of cell death. This happens because of genetic dysfunction that results from a variety of sources, but oftentimes, we cannot be 100% precise in answering the question of why a cancer has developed.

And that is OK; ultimately, we attempt to find ways to help patients despite the uncertainty and deliver the best medical care in their most vulnerable time.

Is Cancer Hereditary?

When we propose that cancer is a genetic disease, we are not implying that the cancer is an inherited disease, passed on from parents to their children, although a minority of cancers are indeed passed along.

Not uncommonly, a patient with cancer would declare to me with clear disappointment, "But no one in my family has ever had cancer," and I would answer, "I know, most cancers are actually not passed along from one generation to another."

It is hard for me to quantify how often the cancer is an "inherited" disease, as this varies based on the cancer itself and the family history. But I have adopted a rule to say that 10% or less of all cancers can be attributed to mutations in inherited genes, and that these mutations are passed along from one generation to another. I would always counsel patients as to whether their cancers might have developed because a gene was passed on from their parents. It's a critical distinction, as it has implications for subsequent offspring. I would argue that the best approach a physician can take to detect the possibility of an inherited cancer is to obtain a detailed family history. Based on that, additional testing might be indicated to determine whether gene mutations were passed along that may have caused the cancer.

So, when someone says cancer is a genetic disease, they really mean that it is caused by genes that control our cells' function and how they grow and divide, like we just discussed. They do not generally mean it is inherited.

Can we screen for some cancers and detect them early? Let's move on to the next chapter.

Take-Home Points

- Cancer can occur in any organ in our body; this makes every cancer different.

- Cancers develop due to an imbalance between cell survival and natural cell death.

- Uncontrollable cell growth and/or lack of natural cell death can lead to cancers.

- This uncontrollable process occurs because of mutations in our genes.

- Mutations can occur because of damage our cells encounter from various factors.

- Some cancers develop because mutated genes are passed from parents to their offspring (hereditary cancers), which happens in the minority of cases.

CHAPTER 2

Screening for Cancer

No amount of experimentation can ever
prove me right; a single experiment can
prove me wrong.

—*Albert Einstein*

MY YOUNG PATIENT, at 56, who was diagnosed with a form of non-Hodgkin lymphoma, walked into my exam room accompanied by his two sons, who were in their early thirties. After discussing the diagnosis and treatment plan, his older son asked me, "What do we need to do now as a family?"

CN: I don't understand the question.

Son: Do we need to get any testing done to make sure that we don't also have the cancer?

CN: No, you really don't. The best thing to do is to support your dad as he goes through treatment.

Son: That we will do. But could we possibly have lymphoma as well? Do we need to get tested?

CN: To my knowledge, this is not a hereditary cancer, and he did not pass anything on to you. Today, we have no definitive evidence that lymphoma has a genetic component that would make it more likely for you to develop it yourselves. But you're likely at a slightly higher risk than the average person because your dad has it. You need regular checkups with your primary doctors and should report any issues or problems you might be encountering. That's all I would recommend.

The son did not seem convinced as he started scrolling through his iPhone screen, consulting Google for the next best testing strategy. He mumbled, "I think we all need to get a PET [positron emission tomography] scan, just in case."

When his dad was getting blood draws, I spent some time explaining that no testing was required. I thought he calmed down a bit; I focused his attention on his dad, but I could understand why he was so nervous, especially as the father of a newborn. He was asking to be screened. He had no symptoms and was feeling well but wanted to be screened "just in case."

As a fellow, I had a gastrointestinal oncology clinic every Monday afternoon and saw a variety of gastrointestinal (GI) malignancies. One patient I saw was a 55-year-old man with colon cancer who came in with his son and daughter. When gathering a detailed medical history, I asked him if he had ever had a colonoscopy prior to his diagnosis. At the time, colonoscopy was recommended to healthy people when they turned 50.

Patient: No, doc. I never had one. I recall my primary mentioning it once, but I got too busy. Now I am worried about my children.

CN: I understand. And your son and daughter will need colonoscopies when they turn 45. Let's focus on your treatment plan now and the next steps.

The year was 1999, and our knowledge of hereditary colon cancers was less mature than it is now. At the time, we would test some cancers to check whether they were related to genes passed on from parents. The universal recommendation was to screen the family members of a patient with colon cancer by doing a colonoscopy when they reach 10 years younger than the age of the diagnosed parent or first-degree relative.

My recommendations for the family of the lymphoma patient were vastly different from my recommendations for the family of the colon cancer patient. But both families were inquiring about screening and what steps they should take to determine whether they were at risk or had already developed the disease.

Screening for cancer essentially requires performing a blood test, imaging study, intervention/procedure, or a combination of thereof in healthy people, with the goal of detecting cancer at an early stage to successfully treat or cure it. The running hypothesis is that detecting cancers early provides patients with a higher chance of cure. Proponents of screening always argue that waiting until a patient has symptoms to look for cancer carries a risk of the cancer being detected too late to be curable. Opponents of screening argue that screening tests are not without risks and could cause complications. Moreover, these tests may detect cancers or other conditions that require no treatment or intervention, as they are not clinically causing any health issues. Indeed, some cancers might not require any intervention, at least when initially diagnosed. In other words, detecting cancers that were never destined to cause any health concerns could lead to harm from unnecessary intervention, increasing the cost of care and causing anxiety for the patient.

Not all screening tests are performed on healthy people. We sometimes screen patients with one form of cancer to check if they have another. A classic example is patients with head and neck cancers with a tobacco use history. These patients are also screened for lung cancer, which, as we know, is commonly associated with smoking.

Of course, the issue with screening is more complex and nuanced than the simplistic view I have provided. There are so many distinctions. Not all cancers have a screening test, and not all tests are equally effective or valuable. Some tests might come back as positive, but the patient has no cancer (we call this a false positive). Other tests might be reported as negative, but the patient indeed has cancer (we call this a false negative). The chances of having a false positive or a false negative result depend on the test, the patient, the cancer being looked at, how prevalent the cancer is in people similar to the patient being tested, the clinical suspicion (before the test is done) of the physician that the patient being tested might indeed have cancer, and other factors. Clearly, there are inherent risks of having false negative or false positive results. If a patient has a false negative, they might not seek medical care and be falsely reassured. If a patient has a false positive, they might undergo unnecessary testing that carries some degree of risk as well.

The universal recommendation across all screening tests is for the patient and physician to have an open discussion and dialogue about these tests and what would be done if the results come back positive or negative. Telling patients beforehand what steps will be taken based on their results will help them decide whether the screening tests align with their views and values. Some patients might choose not to be screened, especially after a certain age, while others might wish to do so. Some physicians might push for screening because of personal bias. It is critical, however, to tailor the screening recommendation based on the patient's goals and beliefs to set proper expectations and ensure appropriate care is delivered.

Screening for Breast Cancer

Few screening tests have gotten the attention mammograms have received over the years. This is partly due to how common breast cancer is in women and because advocacy groups and physicians have pushed for mammography to detect breast cancer early, when it is often curable.

Many medical organizations weighed in on who should be screened for breast cancer, when, and with what. Sometimes these organizations don't see eye to eye, and their recommendations might diverge, confusing patients and their families.

Most medical societies recommend screening women between the ages of 50 and 74 with annual or biannual mammograms. In my experience, most women undergo that test yearly. For women between the ages of 40 and 49, recommendations vary, but most societies agree that women should discuss the pros and cons of the test and be offered a screening mammogram if they so desire. For women over 75, recommendations are not all the same, either. Some propose that evidence for continuing screening at that age is insufficient, while others recommend continued screening as long as the woman is healthy and has no additional medical conditions that might limit her life expectancy.

Pragmatically, what happens in routine clinical practice might not always follow strict guidelines and recommendations. This is related to many factors, but what I have observed throughout my career is that most women are offered yearly screening mammograms starting at age 40.

Years ago, I cared for a young woman who was treated with radiation therapy to her entire chest for her Hodgkin lymphoma, a form of cancer involving the lymph glands. Today, we rarely use radiation therapy to the extent my patient had. Still, the extensive radiation she received put her at risk for developing early breast cancer or other cancers. She received radiation long ago, before the recent advances in radiotherapy, and now we can effectively protect healthy organs from the potentially damaging effects of radiation (see chapter 11 on radiation therapy.) As a result, I asked to see her yearly for a physical and blood work, but also to order some screening tests.

Because of the radiation she received, the common screening guidelines did not apply to her. This underscores the importance of discussing each condition with an expert physician to reach the best screening strategy. In her situation, I recommended magnetic resonance imaging (MRI) of both breasts as she was at greater risk of developing breast cancer than the average woman who has no other risk factors. Because of the radiation's long-term impact on breast tissue, mammograms might not suffice due to scarring. MRIs, however, would improve our ability to find something, if it existed.

But every time we order a test outside of strict guidelines, patients will ask—appropriately so—"Will insurance pay for my test?"

This is a very common but important question. Sometimes, physicians might have to write a detailed explanation of why a woman needs an MRI in addition to a mammogram for screening. This can apply to various types of screening for various types of cancer.

There are other situations where a breast MRI is needed, such as genetic mutations that increase the risk of developing breast cancer; the most well known are the *BRCA1* and *BRCA2* mutations. These mutations put women at a significantly higher risk of developing cancer compared with the general population. An MRI, then, is a better test that can see more than a mammogram can and is therefore a reasonable screening exam for high-risk patients. Another common reason for an MRI is dense breast tissue, where mammograms do not provide adequate imaging clarity. The physician can best determine the ideal screening imaging modality based on these and other factors.

A somewhat new imaging modality is becoming the standard approach for screening women at average risk for breast cancer; it is called *digital mammography* or *tomosynthesis*. Mammograms are two-dimensional, so the radiologist takes two images of the breast: top to bottom and side to side. It turns out that if we take more images from various angles, our detection ability improves. Tomosynthesis permits 11 images during a seven-second exam, allowing it to detect 41% more cancers and reduce the percentage of biopsies and callbacks by 40%. Callbacks mean that the radiologist or the facility will call you back to take more images because they cannot be certain of interpreting what they had seen on the original ones.

Screening for Colorectal Cancer

Colonoscopy has emerged as the best screening test for colon and rectal cancers. The age at which healthy people without symptoms need to be screened has shifted to 45 years.

It is essential to reemphasize here that screening means doing the test on someone who has *no symptoms or abnormal physical exam findings*. If unusual symptoms or findings emerge, the test might need to be performed sooner after consulting with the physician.

A patient of mine had a clear colonoscopy four years before his visit with me. When I saw him, he shared that he had encountered some bloody stools. Further questioning and evaluation made me more suspicious that these were related to something possibly serious. Even though he was not due for another colonoscopy, his symptoms prompted me to move the schedule and send him for an investigative and diagnostic colonoscopy. It was no longer a screening procedure.

This is a salient but critical point. Screening at intervals recommended by the physician is essential, but these intervals are adhered to only if there are no emerging issues or abnormalities. If there are, then patients need to do the doctor's recommended test sooner.

While a colonoscopy is advised at age 45, there are scenarios where this procedure is recommended at earlier ages. Some patients with inflammatory bowel disease (ulcerative colitis and Crohn's disease) and those with hereditary colon cancers (the ones with genetic mutations passed on through generations) might need to be screened much younger than 45.

If you have spoken to friends who have undergone a colonoscopy, they would tell you that the worst part of the procedure is the liquid they must drink the night before to cleanse the bowels so that the GI doctor can clearly see the entire colon and make sure that there are no polyps or growths that need to be biopsied or removed. Most colon cancers develop from *polyps*, which are protrusions from within the inside walls of the colon. If these polyps are removed, cancers are unlikely to develop. Therefore, colonoscopy helps because it can detect polyps that are removed before becoming malignant. Polyps are hypothesized to be more common after the age of 45, which explains in part why screening is recommended at that age. Some colon cancers, however, especially hereditary colon cancers, might not start as polyps, which is one reason these individuals need to be screened sooner.

Other tests have also been recommended to screen for colorectal cancer, such as checking the stools for occult blood (meaning blood you can't see with your eyes). These kits use a chemical called guaiac on a small amount of stool to check for blood. Of course, if there is blood, a colonoscopy is recommended to determine where the blood is coming from.

Some physician policymakers have argued to consider sigmoidoscopy over colonoscopy. The former procedure does not look at the entire colon, just the lower part up to the sigmoid colon; in essence, the scope does not go all the way to the right side of the colon. These physicians argue that doing so, plus checking for occult blood, can save money and still pick up cancers at an early stage. I can see both views, and there are scientific papers arguing each side, but the prevailing point of view today is that screening colonoscopy is the better way to proceed.

There has been some interest in what we call virtual colonoscopy (computed tomography [CT] colonography), which produces images of the entire colon using computers linked to X-rays. If we could do those without drinking that tasteless solution, this test would have taken off. But in my experience, colonoscopies remain the test of choice for most patients who need screening.

A European paper published in the *New England Journal of Medicine* in October 2022 sent the colon cancer community into a heated debate. This paper showed that "recommending" colonoscopy did not reduce mortality. It also showed, however, that the subset of patients who followed the recommendations had less chance of dying from colon cancer.

It is important to discuss with the doctor which tests are recommended and at what frequency. Many physicians propose that no screening is required when the life expectancy is less than 10 years. This does not mean that an 83-year-old woman with abdominal pain should not undergo a colonoscopy (if indicated by the doctor) because the doctor thinks she won't live past 93; rather, because she has symptoms, she will need testing that would no longer be considered a screening test. It is now a diagnostic test that might uncover something treatable.

Screening for Cervical Cancer

The fact that almost all cases of cervical cancer can be attributed to a sexually transmitted virus called HPV makes it a perfect opportunity to screen for and even eradicate. Recall that we discussed in chapter 1 that some cancers are often "caused" by bacteria or viruses, and we can argue that this is one of them.

HPV is considered the most sexually transmitted infection in the United States. The Centers for Disease Control and Prevention (CDC) reported 43 million HPV infections in 2018, mainly among young people. The virus has many types, and not all of them cause cancer. Some can cause genital warts; most HPV infections resolve on their own without causing any health issues. In fact, most HPV infections are transient and do not cause cancers. HPV16 and HPV18 are the two types that cause most cervical cancers.

In addition to cervical and other cancers in the genital areas, HPV has been responsible for some head and neck cancers, especially among patients who have never smoked. Screening methods, however, are available for cervical cancer since women can undergo pap smears. Still, to date, no screening tests exist for head and neck cancers besides routine exams as directed by primary care physicians.

If cervical cancer screening is done periodically, the physician can detect lesions before they become cancerous, and if they are removed, they won't evolve into cancer. Even if they are cancerous, the hope is that the cancer is at a very early stage, where a cure is achievable.

Usually, women undergo pap smears yearly or every other year. The physician determines the frequency related to the patient's age, sexual activity, and family history. In addition, the doctor will check for the presence of HPV and the type of HPV, as not all HPV types are linked to cervical cancer.

You probably know about the HPV vaccine. These vaccines protect against HPV, which helps protect against cervical cancer. HPV vaccinations are therefore essential and recommended for all preteens (including girls and boys), starting at 11 to 12 years old. This protection is not 100%, but it is the best we can do. Thus, vaccinated women should continue undergoing routine cervical cancer screening.

Screening for Prostate Cancer

I once cared for an 82-year-old patient referred to me for his aggressive lymphoma. He was transferred to the University of Chicago from another suburban hospital.

Like all hospital transfers, his came with hundreds of pages of medical records of what happened at the other institution, including all imaging studies and blood tests. While I was mostly concerned about his lymphoma-related studies, I couldn't help but notice that he had a serum prostate-specific antigen (PSA) test as well. I had to ask his wife about it.

CN: Do you know why they checked his PSA?

Wife: No; he usually gets that checked every six months.

CN: Every six months? That's a bit unusual for his age. I know we're concentrating on his current illness, but I ask because I wasn't sure if he had any history of prostate cancer.

Wife: No, he never had prostate cancer; none of his three brothers had prostate cancer or lymphoma, for that matter.

CN: Was he having any problems urinating?

Wife: Not at all.

CN: Thanks; I just wanted to verify the reasoning behind why it was checked.

My patient had a blood test to look for a protein made by prostate cells called PSA. This protein can be produced by normal and cancerous prostate cells. The level of PSA usually increases in men with prostate cancer, although there are other noncancerous reasons why the PSA might be elevated. It can be elevated in men with an enlarged prostate (a common finding as men age) or those with an infected or inflamed prostate.

There is a heated debate about prostate cancer screening. Like other screening tests, the goal here is to find prostate cancer at an early stage, where it can be curable, but sometimes this test can detect a disease that was never destined to cause any health issues. It is not always clear that early detection and treatment decrease the risk of dying from prostate cancer or any other cause, which technically should always be the rationale to perform a screening test. When screening is recommended, a PSA test is usually combined with a digital rectal examination (DRE), where the physician attempts to feel any growths on the prostate gland. A PSA test or a DRE may be able to detect prostate cancer at an early stage, but it is not always clear whether early detection and treatment reduce overall mortality.

Few screening tests are more contentious than a serum PSA for men, partly because it is a quick blood test that was advertised heavily when it became available, but its value remains uncertain. Proponents of PSA screening will always cite graphs of decreased deaths from prostate cancer and attribute that partially to the wide use of that test, which allows them to detect the disease at an earlier stage. Opponents will always contest that finding the disease that early might be an overkill, as some patients never would have lived long enough to develop prostate cancer that indeed requires treatment. In contrast, others might get tested and undergo unnecessary treatments. Treating prostate cancer by removing the prostate can even cause unwelcome complications, including urinary incontinence and impotence.

I have always accompanied my dad to his doctor's appointments. Since he had urinary retention over a decade ago and had to go to the hospital because he couldn't easily pass urine, he became determined to check his PSA often. Every time he had a PSA, it would come back slightly elevated, and I would start worrying about what needed to be done. Is it high because of something serious, or is it just high because his prostate is a bit large, and he is older? He even had prostate biopsies several times because his PSA was high, which all came back negative.

On one of our visits to his primary care doctor, my dad had no complaints except being nervous (as usual) because he was disrobed sitting on the exam table while a nurse's aide was taking his blood pressure. After the examination, his doctor started typing on his keyboard as he documented in the electronic medical records what the visit was about. My dad interrupted the click, click, click of the computer typing:

Dad: Are we going to check my PSA?

Doctor: Do you want to?

Come on, I was screaming inside. *Don't let Dad decide.*

Dad: Yes, of course.

I interrupted: Dad, do you really want a PSA? It was just checked six months ago. What are we going to do with the results?

Dad: Why not do the test and then decide?

Doctor: Well, you're feeling well; we just did the test six months ago, and it was a bit elevated but not concerning. We should either not do it or maybe wait six more months and then discuss.

After a bit more back and forth, my dad agreed, and I triumphed that we avoided unnecessary PSA testing that time. On the next visit, I wasn't so lucky, and he demanded a PSA.

Despite the continued debate on the use of PSA for prostate cancer screening, few would argue against screening when there is a strong family history or a possible hereditary component. Also, the disease is more common in African American men, so screening might be justified even at a younger age in them.

These decisions must be discussed with the physician so that expectations are set before the test is done. "What will we do if it comes back normal, and what will we do if it comes back abnormal?" is an important conversation to have ahead of the test, particularly because most men diagnosed with prostate cancer do not die from it but rather with it, creating the conundrum of what to do when it is detected.

When prostate cancer is detected, likely the first step is to decide whether it is dangerous. Will the cancer threaten someone's life or be a bystander?

I saw a dentist in his mid-sixties with a very mild elevation in his PSA. He underwent a biopsy by his urologist, which showed prostate cancer. His Gleason score was 6.

What is a Gleason score?

When a pathologist looks under the microscope to diagnose prostate cancer, he or she assigns a number representing how distorted these cancer cells are and how vastly different they look from normal cells. If they look very distorted, the pathologist will assign the highest number of 5 (scale is 1–5), and so on. The pathologist looks at the two most common types of cells and assigns two numbers. The combination of these numbers would be the Gleason score, first reported decades ago by Thomas Gleason, a pathologist. Doctors call the distortion I mentioned a grade. So, medically, the Gleason score is calculated by adding the two grades of cancer cells that make up the largest areas of the biopsied tissue sample.

My patient had a Gleason score of 6.

His examination was negative.

"Look," I told him, "you're doing great. Your Gleason score is low; your PSA is low; I feel nothing on the exam. I don't think you need to do anything right now, and we will keep monitoring. Anything we might do could cause side effects, and the treatment could end up worse than the disease," I continued.

You could argue that he should not have had the PSA to start with, but the test was already done, creating the dilemma of what to do next. He was anxious despite my reassurance, and we can't ever underestimate the anxiety that patients experience. We should do what we can to minimize that.

You might hear about other screening tests used for prostate cancer, but none of these are ready for prime time. One that might get done is a urine gene test called *PCA3* RNA, and if it is elevated, urologists might decide on a repeat biopsy. Ultimately, ignore the noise and discuss with your doctor whether PSA and DRE are needed and why.

When prostate cancer is diagnosed early, most patients undergo surgery to remove the prostate gland or radiation therapy that directs beams of radiation to the cancerous prostate. Some patients are observed, like my dentist patient. But these treatments carry risks, so we need to ensure direct and open conversations to address what will be done once the screening results are available.

Screening for Lung Cancer

When I was in training, every attending physician and teacher told me that a classic board question to expect was whether we need to screen for lung cancer. They said that the correct answer was always no. I was taught in the 1990s that no chest X-ray, sputum test, or anything else could detect lung cancer early, even if we do these tests on persons who smoked and have the highest risk of developing the disease.

CT scans, however, have changed what I was taught about detecting lung cancer. A CT scan is a test where the patient lies down in a tunnel-like machine while the inside rotates, taking different X-rays from various angles. The pictures are sent to be analyzed by a computer that creates multiple images showing the tissue, organs, blood vessels, and bones. Helical CT scans offer very thin cuts, so more detailed images of the lungs can be obtained. In the past decade, studies have shown that low-dose helical CT scans can detect lung cancer at a very early stage, a curable stage.

For lung cancer, this was very important as even patients whose cancer is found at the earliest stage possible, when the tumor is localized and has not spread, have a very high risk of recurrence, estimated to be 25%–30%. Proponents of screening use these statistics to make their argument. By now, you should have guessed the counterargument, which is "overdiagnosis" and patients possibly undergoing unnecessary biopsies and testing.

Keep in mind that lung cancer is the leading cause of cancer deaths in both men and women. While a subset of patients who have never smoked develop lung cancer, tobacco use in any form remains the greatest risk factor for developing this disease.

Studies have shown that performing these low-dose CT scans could decrease the risk of dying from lung cancer in heavy smokers. The low-dose CT (sometimes called a spiral CT) uses a very low dose of radiation, so the risk of developing other cancers from these low-dose radiation exposures is minimal. But it is not zero. Therefore, it is essential to make sure that this test is indicated. Initial studies and guidelines recommended screening for *heavy* smokers ages 55 to 74. Why stop at any cutoff age? No one knows. But these original published screening studies had to provide age boundaries because of funding and because we can't have a study that conducts a procedure or an intervention forever. Also, the definition of a heavy smoker can vary; I have yet to ask a smoker if they smoke heavily and hear them concede that they do. In these studies, heavy smoking was defined as one pack of cigarettes per day for 30 years or more (current or ex-smokers). Initial screening studies performed low-dose CT yearly for three years. It is fair to ask if CTs are needed for a longer interval, like mammograms often done annually or every other year. That decision needs to be individualized and discussed with your doctor. This is pertinent especially as the US Preventive Services Task Force (USPSTF) started recommending annual screening for lung cancer with low-dose CT in "adults aged 50 to 80 years who have a 20 pack-year smoking history and currently smoke or have quit in the past 15 years." They further stated that "screening should be discontinued once a person has not smoked for 15 years or develops a health problem that substantially limits life expectancy or the ability or willingness to have curative lung surgery." (A pack-year is defined as number of packs multiplied by number of years. For example, if a person smokes one pack per day for 20 years, it is a 20-pack year; if a person smokes two packs per day for 30 years, it is 60-pack year.)

The biggest issue facing lung cancer screening is that CT findings that might look abnormal on imaging are, in fact, normal. The patient might end up undergoing extensive invasive testing with biopsies or surgeries to know what these findings are. These procedures are not without risks.

Other Screening Tests

I hesitate to write this, but one could argue that getting a physical examination and seeing the general physician periodically is a screening intervention. The doctor might uncover some abnormalities on an exam or learn something from taking a history that leads to discovering something unusual.

I was with my dad during a routine visit to his primary care physician. Dad had no complaints. When his doctor listened to his heart, I noticed he started listening more attentively than usual. He then asked if my dad was drinking too much coffee before his visit, to which my dad replied that he wasn't.

Doctor: Well, I hear a lot of skipped beats; I don't recall hearing that before.

Dad: Is this serious?

Doctor: I hope not, but let's do an electrocardiogram.

An electrocardiogram is a simple test in which some adhesives are placed on the patient's chest and a visual readout of the heartbeat is printed. A few minutes after my dad's test was done, the doctor walked in.

Doctor: I don't really like what I see; you have some changes that suggest high pressures on the right side of your heart.

I knew my dad's blood pressure was now skyrocketing. "Dad, relax," I said. "Let's see what the doctor recommends."

Doctor: Let's do an echo of the heart and assess what is going on.

An echo involves taking pictures of the heart by putting a probe on a patient's chest. This probe transmits images onto a screen, so the technician can see the heart chambers as they move and even the valves that separate these chambers.

The echo documented elevation in the pressures on the right heart chambers, and the doctor then recommended a sleep study. My dad was later diagnosed with sleep apnea and was recommended to wear a device every night when sleeping (called CPAP, continuous positive airway pressure). This eventually normalized his pressures, which likely avoided potentially serious and life-threatening complications.

It was a routine visit, but it led to a diagnosis of a serious problem. True—it wasn't cancer, but I share that story with you to emphasize the importance of maintaining regular visits with primary care physicians.

Another example of how regular visits can help people is skin exams, which doctors perform to detect suspicious pigmentations. My dad was also saved when he saw a doctor who observed something he didn't like on my dad's left forearm and removed it. It turned out to be melanoma, a serious form of skin cancer.

These periodic skin exams, especially in fair-skinned or light-eyed individuals, are critical and can be lifesaving. I always told my patients to be vigilant about any changes in their skin and to share with me any changes in the color or size of their moles. Melanoma can also occur in the eye, so routine eye exams are important, even when vision is not a problem. Keeping a yearly skin cancer checkup on your calendar is always a good idea.

There are other screening tests in rare circumstances, but that is beyond the scope of this chapter.

Informed Decision-Making

There is no perfect screening test, which must be fully explained to people undergoing these examinations. I strongly propose that people should be the drivers in deciding whether to be screened, and I fully recognize that they will rely on their doctor to finalize that decision. I know my dad did. But recall that screening is mainly done in individuals who are healthy and have no symptoms. Therefore, the decision will always be challenging and should never be underestimated.

Patients need to understand the benefits and harms of a screening test. The harms might not lie in the test itself but rather in subsequent testing and procedures that are needed if the test is positive. It is also important to remember that screening tests alone do not diagnose cancer. Any of the screening tests I have mentioned will lead to a cascade of more tests to eventually diagnose or refute cancer as a reason for the findings on the test.

Say a heavy smoker is found to have something on that spiral CT. This "something" that can be a small nodule will need to be biopsied to know if it's cancerous. A biopsy, which requires inserting a needle into the lung tissue, could lead to a punctured lung or other complications. To minimize the risk of screening tests, most healthcare professionals have started developing guidelines that advocate for screening people at the highest risk of developing a particular cancer instead of screening the entire population. I think this is a more sensible approach.

The goal of a screening test is to decrease the chance of dying from the disease being screened for or of dying in general. Sometimes, researchers attempt to quantify whether there is an increase in the number of early-stage cancers found because of screening while the number of late-stage cancers decreases. This observation might be a good reason to consider a screening test. Many will argue, however, that a screening test should not be adopted unless it results in a decrease in overall mortality (death from any cause, and not just the disease being screened for). The controversy over screening will not be resolved entirely in my lifetime.

Take-Home Points

- Screening is doing tests on healthy, asymptomatic people to attempt detecting certain cancers early, when they are at a curable stage.

- The type of screening tests and their frequency differ based on the disease we are screening for.

- It is important to discuss with your doctor whether a screening test is for you before doing the test.

- Some screening tests might fail to detect a cancer that exists (false negative) while others can detect what appears like cancer but is not a cancer (false positive).

- The biggest concern about screening is "overdiagnosis," when we detect cancers that were never destined to cause any problems, but detecting them leads to unnecessary tests that might have side effects and unintended consequences.

- Screening must be a shared decision between the doctor and the patient.

CHAPTER 3

Symptoms and Signs of Cancer

Out of suffering have emerged the strongest souls;
the most massive characters are seared
with scars.

—*Khalil Gibran*

THERE IS NO UNIVERSAL SYMPTOM or sign that leads to a diagnosis of cancer. Moreover, no specific symptom or sign is a definite indication of the type of cancer one might have. Symptoms can happen early or late in the course of a disease and can range in intensity or not even occur at all.

What is a symptom? It is something that a patient feels and believes is unusual and uncharacteristic of that individual. A headache is a symptom. Fatigue is a symptom. Abdominal pain is a symptom.

A sign is something overt that either the patient can witness or the doctor or someone else can observe. If the patient has a fever, that is a sign. If someone notices a patient is yellow or jaundiced, that is a sign. If a patient notices that his urine is darker than usual, that is a sign.

Sometimes these signs or symptoms suggest we are dealing with something profound and life threatening, such as cancer or a heart attack. Other times, they imply something minor, such as a common cold or a tension headache.

It is not uncommon for us to think of the most serious possibility when feeling unwell or having unusual symptoms or signs. We are wired to be concerned, and we often fall victim to the power of suggestion. If a friend was recently diagnosed with cancer, we may be more inclined to think our own unassociated "symptoms" might also be cancer-related.

The best way to describe the signs and symptoms of cancers is by dividing them into three categories.

Signs and Symptoms Based on Location

The signs and symptoms of most cancers depend on where the cancerous tumors are located and, to an extent, on the size of the tumors.

If there is a tumor in the lung, the patient might have a cough, chest pain, or shortness of breath. With the cough, maybe there is phlegm or blood, or perhaps nothing, and it's a dry cough. Someone with a tumor inside the abdomen might develop abdominal pain. If the tumor is large and compresses inside organs, these organs might be damaged and affected, producing additional symptoms. So, some symptoms are related to the impact on adjacent organs. It's also important to note that signs may be related to the location. A tumor in the kidney could cause blood in the urine; a cancer of the colon could cause blood in the stools even when there is no abdominal pain, and so on.

A symptom or a sign alerts the physician that something might be wrong and that a test might be indicated to investigate further. Keep in mind that often, these signs and symptoms are likely not related to cancer at all. As an example, there are many reasons someone could have an enlarged lymph node in their neck: a viral illness, strep throat, an infection, or a benign process. Ultimately, reporting these signs and symptoms to an experienced healthcare professional to sort things out is what I would recommend.

I once cared for a patient diagnosed with colon cancer after she had presented with abdominal pain and blood in her stools. She was doing well and seeing me for a regular checkup after three years of remission. Her husband was with her, and she mentioned that *he* was having abdominal pain similar to her earlier symptoms.

After we conversed a bit, I urged him to see his primary care doctor and get a CT scan. He had a colonoscopy 18 months prior, and my suspicion of colon cancer was negligible. Indeed, he'd had a scan a week later, and his wife called me to tell me that they had found many large lymph nodes inside his abdomen; some were compressing his bowels. Clearly, these large nodes explained his pain. Eventually, he was diagnosed with non-Hodgkin lymphoma that had affected these abdominal nodes. My patient and her husband had identical symptoms of abdominal pain. In fact, that was why she was concerned, because his symptoms reminded her of her own. But in the end, they both had distinctive cancers that would be treated and managed differently.

Another critical note is that symptoms or signs can never tell you the stage of cancer (in chapter 6, I discuss staging extensively). Consider another patient I saw who had presented with a cough and shortness of breath. I decided to do a CT scan of the chest, which showed several nodules in both lungs, one measuring a couple of centimeters. But before doing anything about the lungs, I suggested a CT scan of his abdomen and pelvis. I had a hunch the nodules were originating from somewhere else.

Sure enough, the additional studies showed a kidney mass, and my patient had kidney cancer that had spread to the lungs.

He had presented with chest symptoms, but the origin of the tumor was the kidney. It had spread to the chest, causing the symptoms that made him see me, but the chest symptoms were secondary to the primary cancer.

So, there are no universal symptoms or signs. The location and size of the tumor will cause a symptom or sign. Tests will be ordered to investigate further if the symptoms and signs are related to a serious illness. The take-home message here remains that if you experience something unusual, a consultation with a physician is needed.

General Symptoms and Signs of Cancer

Some cancers can cause generalized symptoms or signs that are not specific to a particular organ's location or the tumor's size. We often call these *generalized symptoms* or *constitutional symptoms and signs*. These can be experienced by anyone with any cancer, although some cancers are more commonly associated with these generalized symptoms and signs than others. The reason these generalized symptoms occur is not known. Some have proposed that the cancer cells can release substances in the blood (proteins or materials related to the body's response to the illness; we call them *cytokines*), and these in turn cause the patient's symptoms.

It's unlikely that I can list all generalized signs and symptoms that can be experienced, but I will highlight the common ones.

Weight loss is an important sign to pay attention to. Of course, we mean unintentional weight loss. If someone is on a strict diet and is trying to lose weight, then weight loss can be a sign of success instead of an ailment. But losing weight without even trying is concerning. This is something that family members or friends might often notice, or the patient might note when clothing becomes too loose and no longer fits. The classic teaching is that we should pay attention to unintentional weight loss of more than 10%. For example, if someone weighing 180 pounds loses 15–20 pounds without trying, there is a cause for concern.

Fatigue is another common generalized symptom that might concern patients and should not be ignored. My approach to fatigue has always been to ask the patient about an example of an activity they used to do but no longer can. This might be the best way to gauge the patient's level and seriousness of fatigue. The activity level is also expected to decrease slightly with age, so putting everything in context is critical. Fatigue is very nonspecific and subjective, so understanding the patient's expectations of their level of activity is important, as often patients might expect that they can do more than they indeed can. I've never forgotten seeing a patient who was in remission from his non-Hodgkin lymphoma but who was concerned that his fatigue could be related to a recurrence or a different cancer.

Patient: I get tired; this was not the case before.

CN: Can you give me an example of something that makes you tired?

Patient: When I walk outside, I get tired.

CN: Well, how long can you walk before you get tired?

Patient: I can walk for 45–60 minutes, but then I need to rest. I can get up the stairs as before.

CN: I don't think this is anything to worry about. But to be sure, we will do routine blood work and ensure that your hemoglobin and thyroid are OK.

I had very little suspicion of anything wrong, but checking his hemoglobin and ensuring he wasn't anemic seemed reasonable. Patients with anemia can feel tired, as red cells are the ones that carry oxygen in the blood to all organs. When the body is short on red cells, patients are labeled anemic, and their ability to carry oxygen all over becomes limited. Hence, they get tired. Low thyroid activity can also cause fatigue, so I decided to check that.

Everything turned out OK, and my patient kept his daily walks, feeling more energized. I couldn't fully explain why he was fatigued, but it could have been due to any variety of life circumstances. Fatigue, for example, can be related to decreased cardiac function, and the patient may need to undergo stress tests. The story's merit is to investigate the cause without assuming that it's always related to cancer, even in a patient with cancer or a cancer survivor. Sometimes, we can't fully explain a symptom, but we must rule out anything serious or life threatening. Occasionally, a symptom reported to an oncologist might not be related to cancer, and referring to another specialist might be needed. I always discuss my suspicion with the primary care physicians and let them determine the next steps once I rule out a cancerous cause.

Fevers and night sweats are generalized symptoms unrelated to a specific organ. The fevers are often low-grade, but if they do not go away in a couple of weeks, this needs to be looked at. The cause of a low-grade and persistent fever might not be cancer, but my point is not to ignore a low-grade temperature that does not resolve with time.

The same applies to night sweats that are unrelated to the weather or the temperature of the room. I mostly get concerned about the "drenching" night sweats. I would ask a patient if they had to change their bed sheets because of the night sweats or if they had to change their clothing because they were drenched in sweat. Also, I get concerned if these sweats do not go away with time. If they happen once and never occur again, I am less concerned.

Pain is often a nonspecific symptom, but it's one that people fear might be related to cancer. Understanding the type of pain (sharp, dull, or a combination of the two), location (all over or at a particular organ or site), frequency (daily, hourly, or once in a while), what brings it on (does it happen at rest, or does activity bring it on?), what takes it away (does it go away on its own or require medication to resolve it, and if so, what kind of medication?), and how long it has been going on (did it just start, or has it been going on for a while and the patient has not voiced a concern until now) can help the physician determine whether the pain is related to a cancerous condition, a noncancerous condition, or something completely benign and not concerning. My point is that no pain, duration, or location is specific enough to signify cancer. So, if there is pain, it is always best to consult the physician and not jump to conclusions.

In my opinion, skin changes can be classified under generalized symptoms and signs. While skin changes can be related to cancer, they are not always related to skin cancer, and sometimes not to cancer at all. Skin that turns yellow can signal something wrong within the liver or bile ducts. But it can also signify a viral infection in the liver. A mole that grows and darkens can signify melanoma skin cancer. Skin changes should be reported to the physician to determine the cause and the next steps.

No Symptoms or Signs of Cancer

Having no symptoms or signs of cancer might sound a bit unusual. How could a life-threatening illness have no signs or symptoms? It can.

As we discussed in chapter 2, the essence of screening is to detect cancers early enough before they start causing any symptoms or signs. That principle implies that cancers could develop without causing symptoms, especially when they are small enough or in their early stages. When we do screening tests, we usually screen for cancers that have not yet caused any symptoms or signs.

Having said that, many cancers may not have symptoms and cannot be screened. An example is a form of non-Hodgkin lymphoma (a cancer that involves the bone marrow and lymph glands called indolent or low-grade non-Hodgkin lymphoma). Many patients with that diagnosis might have no noticeable symptoms at all, and the disease is discovered only when the doctor feels a lymph node or when a patient self-palpates a node. But with an enlarged lymph node, at least a "sign" signifies an abnormality to investigate. There is a form of lymphoma called chronic lymphocytic leukemia (I know it says leukemia, but it is indeed a form of lymphoma), whereby many patients are diagnosed without symptoms when they have routine blood work by their primary doctor.

Also, there are what we call *premalignant conditions*; these conditions are not cancerous yet and have no warning symptoms or signs, but patients who have them are predisposed to cancer progressing from them. For example, some patients with multiple myeloma (a form of cancer involving the bone marrow) have a condition called monoclonal gammopathy of undetermined significance (MGUS), which can sometimes lead to myeloma. Some patients with MGUS, however, may never progress into the cancerous myeloma stage, which is an important nuance.

Take-Home Points

- There is no one symptom or sign that implies a specific cancer diagnosis with 100% certainty.

- Symptoms or signs of any cancer are often related to:

    ◦ Location and size of the tumor.

    ◦ Generalized signs and symptoms that are unrelated to size or location but can occur in many cancers (nonspecific).

- Some cancers have no signs or symptoms. These are often discovered via screening methods that we discussed in chapter 2.

- Unusual symptoms or signs need to be reported to your doctor to determine whether they are related to a severe illness such as cancer, a noncancerous illness, or something completely benign.

- The signs and symptoms cannot determine the origin or the stage of the cancer. These still need to be investigated.

CHAPTER 4

Making a Diagnosis

Medicine is a science of uncertainty
and an art of probability.

—*William Osler*

THERE IS NO SINGLE SYMPTOM or sign that can confirm a cancer diagnosis. Without making a diagnosis, oncologists cannot form a treatment plan or discuss the prognosis with patients and families. The signs and symptoms we reviewed in the previous chapter alert the physician to do more testing to determine what caused them.

These diagnostic tests are procedures used to confirm or exclude a cancer diagnosis, and some can also be used during treatment to determine whether the therapy is working. In most instances, getting a biopsy of the suspicious growth is the gold standard test needed to confirm or exclude cancer.

A biopsy test allows the doctor to get a sample tissue from a suspicious growth. Most commonly, biopsies are done under the direction of radiologists who can localize the area to be sampled, so there is less risk of puncturing the normal tissue. A CT scan or an ultrasound are often done as well to allow better visualization. During the biopsy, the interventional radiologist inserts a needle and takes samples to be examined under the microscope by the pathologist. This outpatient procedure usually requires no hospital stay as long as patients do not encounter complications.

Sometimes, biopsies are done during procedures such as an endoscopy, where the doctor uses a tube inserted in specific organs to visualize their inner parts. For example, a colonoscopy is an exam to visualize the inside of the colon and rectum. If a polyp is found, a sample may be taken, and its pathology report can provide additional information regarding its significance. Bronchoscopy is done to visualize the bronchial tree, the pipes that bring air and oxygen into the lungs. Upper endoscopy is similar in principle to a colonoscopy, but it visualizes the upper gastrointestinal tract (esophagus, stomach, and initial parts of the small intestine). Biopsies of abnormal findings can be performed while doing these procedures. Bone marrow biopsies, a test mainly used when someone is diagnosed with or suspected to have a blood or lymph node cancer, are done to examine the inside of the bone marrow and assess whether a disease is present there. A cystoscopy is an endoscopy test during which a urologist examines the inside of the bladder and its lining. Sometimes, biopsies are done on the skin if the doctor sees an abnormal growth or a suspicious mole.

In certain circumstances, the growth is not accessible with a needle, and patients require general anesthesia and removal of the growth to be examined. We call that a *surgical biopsy*.

Some surgical biopsies require removal of the entire abnormal area, which we call an excisional biopsy. Others are called incisional biopsies, when only parts of the abnormal sites are removed surgically but not the entire abnormality.

Not uncommonly, the tissue sample does not provide a firm diagnosis, and despite best efforts, uncertainty remains.

I recall seeing a patient because of a presumable diagnosis of non-Hodgkin lymphoma. I reviewed the pathology report he brought, and it turns out that he had had a fine needle aspiration, or FNA. An FNA is a type of biopsy that uses a very thin needle and a syringe to remove a sample of cells or fluid from the abnormal area. Generally, an FNA gets less tissue than a true biopsy, and therefore the findings sometimes can be nondiagnostic, meaning no firm diagnosis can be made.

My patient's FNA report stated that the findings were suspicious of lymphoma, so I recommended another biopsy. A suspicious finding is not a solid finding of cancer, so additional testing is warranted.

The testing phase is a time of anxiety and uncertainty. Patients and families want a timely diagnosis to start treatment immediately, but it's important to pause and ensure we are dealing with the *correct* diagnosis. I have taught my students and fellows to explain to patients the importance of additional testing when needed and that waiting a few days is unlikely to change the outcome; instead, it ensures that we are on the right path. I understand, however, how anxious patients can be, and it's important to sit down and explain the details carefully. The bottom line is that when the tissue samples do not provide an accurate diagnosis, performing additional confirmatory diagnostic studies is indicated.

Recently, the term *liquid biopsy* has been used a lot. I will be discussing this in a later chapter in more detail. Briefly, this is a blood test that patients have at a doctor's office, but it is handled differently (in terms of the tubes that it gets collected into, how it is shipped, and so on). The samples are then sent to specialized laboratories where they are checked for DNA, RNA, and/or proteins. This can help determine whether cancer is present or has returned in patients with a known history of cancer who are being monitored.

There are so many other tests that can help diagnose cancer, but, with very few exceptions, none will ever be as confirmatory as an actual biopsy that allows the pathologist to visualize the cancer cells under a microscope. This underscores the role of pathologists in making the diagnosis.

Pathology

According to the College of American Pathologists, pathology is the medical discipline that provides diagnostic information, and it is the discipline that ultimately diagnoses cancer in consultation with clinicians and oncologists.

Once a biopsy is obtained, the pathologist is the physician who determines whether a diagnosis is confirmed or additional testing is needed. Not uncommonly, my colleagues in pathology would call me to advise that additional tissue was needed to finalize a diagnosis. While patients are never happy to undergo yet another procedure, sometimes this is required.

The pathologist performs a vast number of tests depending on the clinical history provided and where the tissue was obtained from. I always taught my students to be as elaborate as possible in providing history and information to the pathologist, as what they do must be put in clinical context.

Once the specimen is received by the pathologist, they will provide a graphic detailed description of what they see (we call this *gross description*), then start performing additional tests. Pathologists and their staff cut thin slices from the tissue to make slides, and they stain these so they can visualize the cells under the microscope. Based on how the cells look and how they are stained, pathologists can often determine their origin. Pathologists explore how the cells are arranged, how distorted they might appear compared with a normal cell, how other features within the cells appear, their size, and other elements. This helps provide initial clues as to what we might be dealing with.

In today's cancer world, additional testing is almost always indicated. Pathologists perform molecular and/or genetic tests that might help them understand the type of mutations the cancer carries, which aids in the diagnosis and potentially in treatment. The pathologist synthesizes all this relevant information before issuing a report concisely describing the condition and finalizing the diagnosis.

A patient was referred to me because of an elevated PSA of 500. The upper limit of normal for that test is about 4; sometimes it goes a bit higher with age, but it should never leap that much in a short window of time. There was little doubt in my mind that the patient had prostate cancer, but I still recommended a biopsy because more information could be obtained from visualizing the actual cells.

Cancer cells can produce substances that can be measured in the blood or urine, raising the suspicion of cancer. These substances are called *tumor markers*. Many types exist, such as CEA for patients with colon cancer and some other tumors; CA19-9 for patients with pancreatic cancer or cancers of the biliary tree; and CA-125 for patients with ovarian cancer. These tumor markers might provide additional diagnostic clues, but by themselves they are largely not considered diagnostic universally. A biopsy remains essential, with few exceptions your doctor can discuss.

Imaging studies also do not diagnose cancer but tell the doctor that cancer may be what causes the pictured findings. Imaging usually helps in staging cancer but is unlikely to confirm its diagnosis. There are so many types of imaging studies that doctors order, but they mainly help us to better understand whether cancer has spread to other areas from where it had originated. I will review more of these in chapter 6, when we discuss staging.

While some patients see the oncologist before a firm diagnosis is made, most are ready for the true first visit once a cancer diagnosis is established.

Take-Home Points

- Performing biopsies of the suspicious growth and obtaining a tissue sample is the gold standard to confirm or exclude a diagnosis of cancer.

- The tissue is sent to a pathologist, who conducts various studies, including molecular and genetic ones, to establish a final diagnosis that is communicated with your doctor.

- Sometimes, a diagnosis cannot be established from the initial biopsy. Additional biopsies might be needed to render a correct diagnosis.

- Patience is needed until your team knows exactly what they are dealing with. Delay for a few days until a final diagnosis is made is better than rushing without certainty about the disease at hand.

- Imaging studies and tumor markers (substances produced by some tumors and detected on blood tests) might provide clues to your team as to what cancer they are dealing with, but with a few exceptions, a biopsy is universally needed.

CHAPTER 5

The First Oncology Visit

The journey of a thousand miles
begins with one step.

—Lao Tzu

THE ANXIETY AND ANTICIPATION of that first oncology visit cannot be overstated. By the time your appointment is made, so much has been done—likely some imaging studies, biopsies, asking family and friends about your diagnosis, and a lot of googling. Most patients see the oncologist that was recommended by their primary care physician or their surgeon, and that's excellent, but it never hurts to ask around and investigate. Maybe someone you know—a relative, a colleague, or a neighbor—has heard of the doctor you'll be seeing. Word of mouth is important. What you need, in addition to someone who is knowledgeable in the field, is someone attentive, available, and communicative with you and your loved ones. Sure, many patients gravitate toward oncologists who have lectured a lot, written so many articles on the topic, and are thought leaders, but that doesn't always translate into empathy and compassion. I believe that these last two traits are critical, as the journey of this disease is filled with bumps, and you want someone who can help you navigate the uncertainties and shepherd you as you both develop a cohesive management plan.

The newly diagnosed cancer patient is likely to want to see a specialist right away. You were just told you have cancer, and we can all agree that with a few exceptions, any cancer diagnosis is traumatizing. But for more than 95% of cancers, seeing the oncologist is not an emergency, so if your appointment is a week or two away, don't panic; instead, use that time to gather more information and prepare for your first visit. If your doctor senses that this is an emergency, they will admit you to the hospital to have you seen and expedite the process. That only happens when the doctor feels that starting treatment for the diagnosed cancer simply cannot wait. In those cases, you will be informed of the need for immediate care. So, to the best of your ability, follow your doctor's lead in terms of the timetable.

While waiting for the appointment, my suggestion is to do the following:

- **Read about your cancer:** Sure, there is a lot of bad information on the internet, but there is a lot of important and accurate information out there too. Always consider the source. I'd suggest visiting websites of reputable cancer centers in your area, such as the American Cancer Society website, or the National Cancer Institute. Educating yourself about the disease is essential; it allows you to be your own advocate, and if a doctor is intimidated by you researching the disease or feels uncomfortable with your knowledge, this is not the doctor for you. Oncologists must embrace patients' own advocacy and should encourage patients to research and be educated. I did that throughout my career, but I was picky about where my patients got their information. If you find an article or two that are intriguing, you should bring them to your first visit. This self-education will generate questions that you need to write in a notebook or your phone or tablet for later reference. I'll share with you later a list of questions that you'll want to ask during your first visit.

- **Prepare your medical history**: There should be no doubt that your doctor has already received much of your records. These records may not be complete, but at a minimum, your oncologist likely knows the type of cancer you have. Sometimes, patients are referred to the oncologist to ensure they don't have cancer, but that's the minority of cases. Your oncologist hopefully has access to medical records available in the hospital where you were originally seen, but as you'll learn later, if you are seeing someone for a second opinion, these records are not always complete. If you have records from a different hospital or from a different system, you'll need to bring these with you. So, prepare whatever records you possess to give to the doctor when you visit. Consider writing on a piece of paper when you started having symptoms, when you had certain procedures, and whatever else you were going through. You may even want someone with you at your appointments: your spouse, a trusted friend or a family member, or someone else who can take notes and ask questions. Your oncologist will take a detailed history, and while you have probably told your story to many other professionals before seeing the oncologist, you'll need to do it one more time. This one is so important, as the nuances and details of every history can have important implications. Don't hold back, be honest, and provide all the information. In summary, bring all the records you have and, better yet, summarize the sequence of events that led to your diagnosis as well. You're about to meet your teammate in this journey, and they need to know the details to move forward and formulate a plan.

- **Bring your medications**: Bring all your medications with you. Oftentimes, patients forget to bring whatever nonprescription supplements they're consuming. Your doctor needs to know everything you're taking as some of what you might think is totally benign can interact adversely with a medication your oncologist will prescribe. Be inclusive and comprehensive. Whatever vitamins, herbs, and supplements you've been taking are all important for your oncologist to know.

• **Develop coping skills:** There is no doubt that the coping process starts at the time of suspecting you might have cancer. I once had a CT scan on my abdomen as I was having some unusual pains. I recall how anxious I was as I waited for the results. I was making mind calculations as to what the diagnosis might be and what I would and wouldn't do if there was cancer. I am sure you felt the same for a few weeks before your first visit. The need to cope with the diagnosis heightens when it is confirmed, and as you wait for that first visit, you need to find ways to minimize the rising stress level that is understandable and expected. The word "cancer" can make you feel helpless and scared, and give you a sense of loss of control. These are all normal reactions to a stressful event. But there are things you can do to help mitigate the stress and anxiety you may be feeling. If you meditate, that is great, and you should keep doing so. If you don't, try it a few times; it does help. I recommend you go for walks with a loved one or a dear friend. It is OK to talk about how you feel with trusted friends or family. If you can exercise a bit, that can help. If you are struggling with anxiety or depression, seeking a good therapist can be a tremendous help; having professional mental health support can make the cancer care journey easier to bear.

• **Share the diagnosis:** This is a very personal decision. Most of my patients waited a bit before telling extended family members and friends, as they expected to be bombarded with questions that they might have no answers to until after the initial oncology visit. No matter what, I recommend never going to the first oncology visit alone. Bring someone you trust who can provide another set of ears in case you miss some of the conversation. Being overwhelmed is expected, and having someone with you to take notes and ask more questions is optimal. Identify at least one individual to do this. Going together to the first oncology visit is something I cannot overemphasize. Every time I saw a patient alone for their first visit, I wanted to know why. Understanding that piece helped me gain more knowledge about the patient and their family dynamics. All these elements can prove useful when deciding on a treatment plan and the next steps.

Sharing the diagnosis with your place of employment is a different story. My advice is to wait until you know the plan. Your employer likely would want to know whether you need fewer work hours, more days off, or other arrangements. You're unlikely to have these answers until after you consult with the oncologist. Recall that some cancers might need surgery and others might require no therapy. Waiting until you're armed with more information is wise because it allows you to provide a more complete picture of the situation to relevant parties. Some patients like to share their stories on social media; this might allow you to connect with like-minded people who can help you along the journey. Others might be more private and reserved, not wanting to use social media for this purpose. This is another personal decision that I don't feel strongly about. I just want you to know that social media is another resource that you can use however you see fit but be wary of some information out there; it is not reviewed by medical professionals, and anyone can post whatever they want, regardless of accuracy.

- **Check your insurance:** Once you have your diagnosis, you may want to call your insurance carrier to go over coverage and necessary documentation. Most oncologists have administrative staff who will check your responsibility, but I recommend you also do that yourself. It might generate questions that you will want to ask your oncologist when you visit.

Your First Oncology Visit Day

Your appointment day is here; I don't want you to go alone. What should you expect when you get to the oncologist's office, and what type of questions must you ask? In some academic centers, you may be seen by a medical student, a resident, or a fellow before you see the attending oncologist who is ultimately responsible for your case. Don't let that surprise you, and remember that even the best oncologists and the most famous doctor you've ever heard of were once students, residents, and fellows. These trainees will not make the ultimate treatment decision, but they will observe and learn from the attending physician how to approach a case so they can become independent in a few years. Be courteous and responsive to their questions; they're part of the team, and rest assured that their involvement is not affecting your care adversely. In fact, it is likely going to help. In some oncology settings, you may be seen first by a nurse practitioner or a physician assistant, collectively labeled as advanced practice providers, or APPs. The APPs are also integral members of your care team, and they're helping the oncologist with follow-up tests, procedures at times, and seeing new patients and follow-ups. The bottom line is that whoever sees you is part of the team and is there to help care for you.

- The oncologist is going to ask you questions that you have answered many times before. You're expected to walk the oncologist through your story and what has happened. That is where the summary page I advised you to make can come in handy because it aids in understanding the continuity of the story.

- The oncologist and care team are going to conduct a physical examination. Some elements of the exam might differ based on the diagnosis.

- The oncologist will want to know more about you, the person behind the disease. What are your goals and values? These are important to share as they might direct some of the treatment decisions. What are your needs? What is on your mind, and what is generating fear and anxiety? Oncologists might want to know about your hobbies, daily activities, interests, work, and family dynamics. All of these are essential considerations moving forward.

- The oncologist is then expected to review the findings with you and spend some time explaining the diagnosis and whether additional tests are needed and why. Take notes and have your family or friends who are with you take notes as well. I have had patients record me when I was sharing information, and that is OK. But please ask permission. Doctors should be OK with that if you ask beforehand. You need to grasp what is being explained to you, and sometimes listening to this later helps. The most helpful part is having another set of ears in the room. In my view, that is better and more important that any notes or recordings you might take.

- After all this information gathering and discussion, there are several possibilities regarding next steps:
  - Your oncologist formulates a treatment plan and discusses it with you during the first visit.
  - Your oncologist needs additional testing (see chapter 6) to stage your disease and then decide on a proper treatment plan.
  - Your oncologist has some idea of what is best but wants to discuss your case with colleagues who are familiar with your type of cancer. Many hospitals and cancer centers have what we call tumor boards. These are conferences where various cancer specialists gather to discuss cancer cases that require involvement of more than one doctor or cases that are challenging to make a treatment decision. Ask your doctor when your

case will be presented and when you will receive the feedback and recommendations.

- It is possible that the diagnosis you came in for is not final, and your oncologist might suggest more biopsies.

• If a treatment is decided upon during your first visit, logistics of the therapy will also be discussed. The pros and cons and potential side effects and how these are managed will also be discussed. Prognosis might also be discussed during the first visit, although most oncologists wait until they see how patients respond to a therapy.

• Here is a list of questions to ask your oncologist during your first visit. Not all of these questions will be applicable to you, but many will be. Be prepared to take notes, and ask whomever you've invited along to also take notes and ask questions.

- What is my exact diagnosis?
- Is this the type of cancer that occurs in my age group, or is this unusual?
- Did I get this cancer from my parents? Could I have passed it on to my family members or children? Should we have genetic testing done?
- What stage is my disease? If we don't know the stage, what tests do I need to know the stage?
- Is my disease curable?
- What are my options for curing the disease?
- How long do I need to stay on therapy? How often is it given and for how long each time?
- Can I still work full-time while getting my treatment?
- Are there restrictions at work if I stay full or part time?
- Should I take a medical leave?
- Do I need a family member or a friend caring for me at all times?

o Do I need to take time off school? If so, when can I go back?
o What are the side effects of the recommended treatment? How common are they, and how often do they occur? What bodily changes should I expect?
o What strategies do we have to counter and mitigate these side effects?
o Are any of the side effects potentially permanent, or do they reverse once we complete treatment?
o Does the treatment impact fertility? Can anything be done about that?
o Do you think my mood will be affected?
o If we can't cure my cancer, what can we do about it to slow its growth?
o Can you tell me about my prognosis?
o Should I enroll in a clinical trial?
o Is it OK if I get a second opinion? Will you help me in doing so?
o Can you give me any resources so I can learn more about the disease?
o Do you recommend any support groups for me and my loved ones?
o How do I reach you during business hours and after hours? If something happens, who do I reach out to first?
o How will the cancer affect my relationships with my friends, family, and significant other?
o Will my cancer or its treatment affect my ability to have sex?
o Should I tell my extended family members I have cancer?
o What activities should I avoid?

The first visit is one of many to follow, but it is critical as it establishes the initial rapport you need to have with your doctor. Trust your instinct. Do you feel comfortable with the oncologist's demeanor, answers, responsiveness, bedside manner, and office staff? You're about to embark on a journey, and you need the right team to guide you and be there with you every step of the way.

Take-Home Points

- As you wait for your first oncology visit, prepare by collecting your medical records (especially for second opinions), gathering all your medications (including over-the-counter, or OTC, medications), finding ways to cope (talk to friends, meditate, exercise, walk, or seek counseling if needed), and identifying a trusted family member or friend to be with you during this first visit.

- Research your disease from trusted websites and sources.

- Sharing your diagnosis with your extended family members or broadly on social media is an individual decision.

- Sharing with your employer is important, but timing is best after you know more about the disease and plan.

- Do your best not to go to your first oncology visit alone.

- Bring a notebook, and write down answers to questions provided in this chapter.

CHAPTER 6

Cancer Staging

Everything should be made as simple
as possible, but not simpler.

—*Albert Einstein*

TO DECIDE ON PROPER TREATMENT and the best approach,
knowing the extent of the cancer in the body is critical. This process
is called *staging*.

I recall seeing a patient years ago. He had a disease called chronic
lymphocytic leukemia, or CLL. As to be expected, one of his questions was, "What is the stage of my cancer, doc?" I told him it was
stage 0, and his jaw dropped.

"What do you mean by stage 0; do I not have cancer?"

"Yes, you do," I responded empathetically. "It's just that this type
of cancer is staged from 0 to 4, and we have been using that staging
system since 1975."

"When do I get my CT scans?" he asked. "I read that I need scans
to know where the cancer might have spread."

"You actually don't need scans at this point to stage your disease;
we stage it by doing blood tests and physical exams."

I felt I was losing my patient and that he was ready to go see someone else. I continued, "Every cancer is staged differently. Let me tell you more about CLL and what we mean when we stage it."

Basically, all patients are familiar with the term "staging." Often, they associate it with numbers, and the higher the number, the worse the prognosis. Every patient knows that stage 4 is worse than stage 3, which is worse than stage 2. It is engraved in our brains somehow to aim for the smaller number when it comes to staging.

But that is a bit too simplistic and frankly, not even accurate. I remember seeing a patient with a form of leukemia, called acute myeloid leukemia (AML). In that disease, cancer cells that are generated from the bone marrow (think the factory that produces all blood cells in our body) circulate in the blood. How can we stage a cancer that circulates in the blood and streams all over our body? My patient wondered if he had stage 4 because the cancer cells were in the blood, and I tried to explain that blood cancers are a different beast and are staged and treated differently.

When I was at the University of Chicago, I was asked by my department chair to cover the head and neck cancer clinic for a few months. The anatomy of the head and neck region is rather complex, so I started refreshing my memory on staging this disease and its therapies. I quickly learned that there are patients with stage 4 disease (technically the highest number you can get) who can be cured. How could that be? I bet that when most patients hear "stage 4," curing the cancer never crosses their minds.

One of my relatives developed colon cancer. He had encountered a few bouts of bloody stools, and a colonoscopy detected a cancerous growth in his colon. When his doctor ordered CT scans, these showed an additional growth in the liver. There was no cancer anywhere else in his body. He called me asking my opinion and what I thought his stage was.

"Well, unfortunately, it is stage 4," I said.

"How many stages are there?" he asked.

"There are four stages of colon cancer."

"So, that's it?"

"No; it's not; we have many treatments for colon cancer, and they are very effective. Also, if we get lucky and can remove the growth from your liver, there is a chance that we could cure your cancer." I continued to explain that a minority of patients with stage 4 disease like the one he had could be cured.

My relative was not convinced. "How can my disease be stage 4 and still be cured?" he asked. "I should have checked Google," he said as he managed a faint smile. We were conversing on Facetime, so I could see his facial expressions and how his skin had paled from the anemia.

He contested that he had joined a colon cancer support group, and patients with stage 4 he had met had incurable disease.

I spent some time explaining to him that some patients with stage 4 colon cancer can indeed be cured. Not all advanced-stage disease is incurable. I asked him not to compare his condition with that of others, as every situation is different, and the devil is in the details. I promised him that I would help him every step of the way as he navigated this disease with his oncologist, who specialized in managing colon cancers.

Few people are unfamiliar with Lance Armstrong, the American cyclist who was stripped of his consecutive Tour de France wins due to doping and using performance-enhancing substances. One other aspect of Lance's life that is well publicized is his cancer story. On October 2, 1996, Armstrong was diagnosed with testicular cancer that had spread to his brain. He was treated with surgery by removing the affected testicle, followed by chemotherapy. He also had surgery to remove the two cancerous brain tumors. He recovered, and the cancer never came back. Lance then founded the Lance Armstrong Foundation (which later became the Livestrong Foundation) to assist other cancer survivors. Most lay people would not have guessed that a cancer that goes to the brain could be cured.

Staging refers to the extent of cancer in someone's body. The staging process can be complex and cumbersome for patients. It is certainly one of the areas that generates the most anxiety and concerns, especially as patients wait for test results that are destined to determine their stage. On one hand, receiving a diagnosis of cancer is life altering by itself, but on the other hand, knowing the extent of the disease is a whole other ball game.

There is no universal approach to staging. Essentially, physicians use various types of imaging and laboratory studies to determine whether the cancer has spread or has remained in the area of origin. But how we stage each cancer depends on the cancer itself. So, if you know someone who had undergone different studies to stage their cancer than the ones you did, it doesn't mean your doctor is doing anything wrong. You simply have two different cancers.

The way we should approach staging is by separating blood cancers (some patients and physicians call these *liquid tumors*) and other cancers that originate from solid organs. Discussing the staging procedures with the oncologist is critical as there is no universal approach to staging all cancers.

In rectal cancer, for example, endoscopic ultrasound (a minimally invasive procedure that introduces a special endoscope through the rectum that uses high-frequency sound waves to assess the lining and walls of the rectal area) has become an important procedure of the staging process since it allows the endoscopist to visualize the depth of the tumor infiltration into the bowel wall. That depth does affect prognosis and what therapy the medical team will prescribe. In lung cancer, physicians order a brain MRI because some patients have disease spread to their brains despite having no symptoms. The chances of that happening vary based on the type of lung cancer, but the percentage of patients who have occult brain metastases is high enough to justify looking for it. We don't do that routinely in patients with lymphoma or breast cancer, for example, unless there are symptoms that warrant doing the imaging study.

In general, there are some standard staging imaging studies (usually CT scans) to be performed for most cancers and additional studies dictated by the patient's symptoms, such as a brain MRI in someone with cancer who has unexplained headaches. These are supplemented by more studies that are dictated by the cancer itself, similar to the few examples I mentioned. The collection of all this information determines the stage of the cancer.

But I am still not convinced how all this complex information and variation in staging based on the disease helps simplify patients' understanding of their stage. How does knowing the stage number resonate with patients and families, and how much does it indeed matter?

When I started seeing patients as a faculty attending, one of my goals was to make sure my patients and their families understood what we were dealing with. I often would pause midsentence and ask them to recount what we had just discussed. With time, I started refining my explanations based on my observations of what confused patients the most. Staging was certainly one of these topics.

I became increasingly dissatisfied with the idea of staging cancers from 1 to 4, or from 0 to 6, or whatever number there was. Such a staging system is helpful for academicians and scientists so that we can compare apples to apples and so that when we discuss clinical trials, everyone is speaking the same language. From a patient perspective, however, I was not convinced it was that helpful.

In my opinion, every cancer, whether blood cancer or a solid tumor, has two stages and two stages only. It is either the curable stage or the controllable stage. The controllable stage can eventually progress to a noncontrollable one, which some might label as terminal, although that definition is not one of my favorites. When a patient presents with any kind of cancer and they ask for the stage, they're really asking whether the cancer is in a stage that can be cured or not. Whatever number we stamp on that cancer matters less from a patient perspective. Some cancers start in a curative stage, but their course might shift to the controllable one. I started asking my patients if they cared more about the stage number or about the goals of therapy, and universally the answer was the latter.

When I started explaining the stage to my patients using the format of "curable versus controllable," I sensed that they understood the condition better; they related easier. Telling a stage 4 head and neck cancer patient that they had stage 4 created panic and helplessness, but saying to that same patient that they had a potentially curable stage created hope and more realism. That doesn't mean we can't say both, but it means that we need to refine our medical language to ensure that our patients understand what we are doing and that they have simplified answers to a complex condition.

Most patients with prostate cancer that I had cared for had a disease that had spread elsewhere, and cure was not an option.

I recall a patient who was a retired physician and who was seeing me for a second opinion. His disease had started in the prostate but spread to his bones. He was accompanied by his wife, and we were discussing his stage.

"I have stage 4; it's terminal," he announced.

"Why do you say terminal, and what do you mean by that word?" I asked.

"Because it's going to kill me. I have stage 4 cancer."

"Let's not talk numbers," I suggested. "You have a prostate cancer that is in a controllable stage. It is not curable, but it is controllable."

"I don't understand." He sounded confused, but his wife started taking notes.

"Look. You do have diabetes and a blood pressure problem, don't you?" I asked, knowing the answer. "Neither of them is curable, but you do take medications for both, and they are both controlled." I continued, "Your prostate cancer is in a similar stage. We can't get rid of it just like we can't get rid of your hypertension or diabetes, but we can control it, and we will." I was looking him in the eyes, making sure he heard every word I was saying.

We discussed how we would control his prostate cancer and what treatments he would receive. He no longer was interested in whether he had stage 3 or 4, but he did want to know how long we could control his cancer. I explained to him my prediction and that it could change based on how he responded to various therapies he received.

Even pancreatic cancer, which is viewed as one of the most ominous cancers, is potentially curable. Obviously, the percentage of cure and control vary based on a host of factors related to the disease itself and to the patient.

With time, I shifted the way I discussed staging with all my patients to explaining the "two-stage" approach. I even taught my residents, students, and fellows as such. One of my mentees that I trained, and who is now practicing oncology in the south side of Chicago, texted me out of the blue one day thanking me for teaching her how to discuss staging with patients.

"It really resonates well," she said.

"I am glad I could help," I replied. "Ultimately, our goal is to explain processes from a patient's perspective. We're not writing an academic paper when we're in the exam room trying to deal with a life-altering event."

"Only two stages to every cancer," her text read with a smiley emoji.

Another way to stage solid tumor cancers is based on whether they are localized (located only in the original organ), regional (in the organ plus close by lymph nodes), or systemic (has spread to distant areas in the body beyond where it originated). Despite the fact that I have always used the curable versus controllable staging approach, physicians and textbooks of course will always use the traditional method of staging by numbers, which is important as we discussed above. Even when the number staging is used, don't hesitate to ask, "Do I have a curable or a controllable stage?" If it is the curable stage, ask how it will be cured, and if it is the controllable stage, ask how it will be controlled. Sometimes, we know from the get-go whether a disease can be cured or only controlled. As I stated above, in some circumstances, the controlled cancers can become uncontrollable when our treatments are no longer effective.

In the end, a simple explanation from a patient angle is what matters.

As far as what tests are needed to know whether a patient has a curable or a controllable stage, there are many, and as I mentioned, deciding which ones to do depends on the disease, the patient, the goals of therapy, and the clinical condition. Here are the common tests:

- **CT scan:** This is a donut-shaped X-ray machine that is linked to a computer to take various pictures of the inside of the body from different angles. Some scans require a contrast material that gets injected in the vein, as well as a different kind of dye that gets swallowed. Some scans are done without these. Your doctor decides whether you need contrast based on what they're looking for. Rarely, patients might have an allergy to the contrast, and if you do, your doctor will give you medications before you receive the dye, to prevent bad reactions. The modern CT scan machines take continuous pictures in a helical or spiral fashion rather than individual slices. The process requires you to lie on a table that passes through the center of the machine. You might hear noises during the procedure, and the technician will likely ask you to hold your breath every so often while you are being scanned. The procedure causes no pain, but you may be a bit uncomfortable lying on your back. The entire process should be completed in less than 30 minutes. There is some radiation exposure when undergoing CT scans, so pregnant women are not recommended to have the test done. You might have heard about the risk of developing cancers from radiation exposure, but the risk of developing any cancer from CT scans is very small, and it is far more important to know the extent of the cancer to guide treatment.

- **MRI**: MRI is another imaging study where you lie on a table that is pushed into a long, round chamber. This machine makes loud noises and rhythmic beats, so the technician will put headphones on your ears and may let you listen to your choice of music. The MRI uses a powerful magnet and radio waves to take pictures of the body. It is particularly good for brain and spine imaging. Usually, the MRI requires a contrast injection by vein that is different from the CT scan contrast. It is called gadolinium.

- **Bone scan**: This test specifically assesses whether the bones are involved with cancer. It is what we call a *nuclear test*, in which a small amount of a radioactive material is injected into the vein. This material accumulates in abnormal areas of bones. Some of these areas can be related to cancer, but not every abnormal bone scan is indicative of cancer. The abnormal areas appear dark on the imaging study, and we call them *hot spots*. Bone scans are done for some but not all cancers. As an example, they are often ordered in prostate cancer but not in rectal cancer.

- **PET scan**: A PET scan is another nuclear test in which a small amount of radioactive material (glucose or sugar) is injected into the vein. The computerized images of the areas show where the glucose is taken up by various parts of the body. Theoretically, cancer cells take up more glucose than normal cells, so the obtained pictures can show the areas where there is more sugar uptake, suggestive of possible cancer, although other processes such as inflammation can sometimes show similar pictures. The PET/ CT study uses the PET scan and CT scan imaging in one procedure. The CT scan is done first to help define the anatomical structures. This is followed by the PET scan, which shows the active areas, or what we call *functional* or *hot*. Doing these two studies together provides more accurate information on tumor location and possible spread. It also can reduce the number of imaging procedures done. What we need to remember is that some cancer cells might not take up sugar like others, so the PET images in these cancers might be less informative. An example is kidney cancer, where a PET scan has not been routinely performed.

- **Ultrasound**: This procedure uses high-energy sound waves to look at internal organs. We see these images on a computer screen. I'd say these are more helpful when trying to locate a tumor to biopsy, but not to do a comprehensive staging. The patient lies on a table during the exam and the tech moves a transducer (a device that transforms one form of energy to another) on the skin over the body parts that are being visualized. The tech will use a cold gel on your skin that makes the visualization better and easier.

- **Routine X-rays**: X-rays generally don't help in staging, and certainly more sophisticated studies are needed. They do, however, have a role in addition to other staging modalities. For example, we often do X-rays of the entire skeleton in patients with multiple myeloma, a cancer of the bone marrow. Doing X-rays of the skeleton in myeloma can help the clinician to decide on the need for treatment in certain circumstances.

- **Bone marrow biopsy**: In liquid tumors, we often need to assess whether the cancer cells have gone inside the bone marrow. Usually, a needle is inserted inside the iliac bone (hip bone) and the marrow is aspirated (meaning the needle withdraws some of the marrow's fluid). A piece of bone is taken as well. The liquid and bone are both examined under the microscope, and additional sophisticated studies are done to detect any cancer cells.

One of my most memorable patient visits was with someone I saw for a second opinion. She was diagnosed with lung cancer when a growth was found on the left side of the lungs, but there was also a growth on her left adrenal gland—a gland atop the kidney that is critical for hormonal balance in the body.

She arrived and announced that her chemotherapy would begin the following week. But I suggested that surgery to remove both growths might actually do more to cure her cancer than chemotherapy alone.

"But I didn't think it was curable. It's stage 4," she suggested.

"Yes, it is," I responded, "but that doesn't mean we can't try to cure it. It simply means that the cancer has spread to other locations. Still, the tumors are local to the lung and the adrenal gland, so we might have a chance for a cure if we operate."

She was concerned about her age (72) being an impediment to successful surgery, but after reassuring her that we would run tests before deciding on that route, she seemed eager to try.

After extensive evaluation, my patient underwent surgery, and she had both growths removed. She then received chemotherapy for a few months. I received a greeting card from her as I was leaving the University of Chicago, wishing me well. I smiled as I read it and was beyond elated that she continued to do well. This story and many others have emphasized to me that one hat never fits all. Fast forward, however, and nowadays it is not uncommon to start with chemotherapy before surgery for lung cancer in scenarios like my patient.

In summary, there are so many tests your doctor can order, but they will tailor which ones to use based on your particular disease. After the results of these tests become available, your doctor should hopefully be able to communicate with you the stage of your cancer and whether it is a curable or a controllable stage. This will help determine the treatment plan. As these plans are being discussed with you, should you consider a second opinion? Should you explore clinical trials? I will discuss these questions next.

Take-Home Points

- Staging is assessing the extent of cancer in the body.

- Every type of cancer can be staged differently with different set of tests that are ordered by the doctor and dictated by the type of cancer.

- Academically, doctors use a staging system with numbers; the higher the number, the worse the stage.

- From a patient's perspective, it is easier to divide stages into:

    ○ Curative stage: cancers that we think we can cure when we diagnose them.

    ○ Controllable stage: cancers that we know we cannot cure at the time of diagnosis. Some cancers start in a curable stage but move into a controllable stage if they recur. The ability to control a cancer might wane with time, and the cancer can become uncontrollable.

CHAPTER 7

Second Opinions

When you want something, all the universe
conspires in helping you to achieve it.

—*Paulo Coelho*

MY PATIENT AND HER HUSBAND—a physician—sat across
the room from me. She had advanced-stage cancer that was not curable but was potentially controllable. As I explained the situation, she
became emotional, understandably so, and said, "There is no way this
is true; we must cure this."

"We definitely have the means to control it and hopefully for many
years to come," I explained, "but I don't see us getting rid of it completely. It has gone to other organs." Unlike my earlier patient with
the adrenal growth, this patient had growths in various areas where
surgery was not an option.

"I want a second opinion," she said firmly and immediately.

I gave her a few names and told her that I would help her get an
appointment after she decided whom she wanted to see. I also asked
my staff to make copies of her medical records so that she could take
those along with her.

My patient's condition was very straightforward from an oncology standpoint. It would be unimaginable that any oncologist would suggest a cure, but she was unhappy with my statement and felt that seeing someone else to discuss it was in her best interest. My goal was to ensure that she saw whomever she needed to so that she could proceed with the proper choice, whether with me or someone else. I did ask myself whether her decision was because of something I said or the way I said it, but in the end, I supported her decision.

One of the lymphoma patients I saw lived 50 miles away from the medical center where I practiced. He had an early stage disease that required a few cycles of chemotherapy. He came to see me for a second opinion after his doctor made the proper recommendations. After I concurred with the recommendations provided by his local oncologist, I urged him to go back and get his care under her direction. I told him that driving 50 miles back and forth every time he needed chemotherapy was not necessary and that he might require interim visits along the way. He was thankful and continued to see me periodically while getting his care closer to home.

Another patient came in to see me accompanied by his extended family. He was in a wheelchair as his cancer and treatments had taken a toll on him. He was coming for a second opinion after his local doctors had recommended no further therapy. Instead, they suggested focusing on symptom management under the hospice umbrella. In reviewing his records and prior therapies, it was evident that he had no viable options, including experimental therapies for his disease. After discussing the condition, I explained to him and his family why my recommendations mirrored those of his local doctors.

I knew that he had come in for a second opinion hoping that it would differ from the prior opinions he had received. I wanted to disagree with his doctors and offer him something fruitful. In the end, the second opinion was similar to the first.

One patient I saw for a second opinion was self-referred. He was diagnosed with an indolent form of non-Hodgkin lymphoma, called follicular lymphoma, and his doctors had recommended no treatment as he was having no symptoms.

When I saw him, I advised that this recommendation was reasonable but that I needed to see the pathology slides to ensure that my team and I agreed with the diagnosis. Upon review, we were able to see the follicular element, but our findings suggested that he had a more aggressive form of this cancer than had been appreciated. My recommendation was therefore chemotherapy. I called the primary oncologist and explained our findings and advised the patient that sometimes these discrepancies occur. Understandably, the patient was not too thrilled that there was significant divergence in opinion as he wanted to hear the same recommendation. He was served well by undergoing the chemotherapy that cured his lymphoma eventually.

Some patients seek a second opinion wishing to hear the same opinion they received, while others (like my patient who was referred to hospice) seek another opinion hoping they hear a different recommendation. What is critical is to always offer a new opinion based on independent evaluation and not to be affected or influenced by what others might have recommended. This might be easier said than done, however.

When seeing patients, it was important to me to tell them that it was totally OK to seek another opinion. It became part of how I concluded my first consultation visit with them. I also taught my fellows and students to do the same. Patients often think about getting a second opinion, but they might be embarrassed to ask or declare what they want to do. Taking that fear away and affirming that this desire is normal deepens the trust between the oncologist and the patient. A typical end to a patient visit would be me saying: "I know there was a lot that we discussed today, and I am always here to explain further. It is not uncommon that you might want to get a second opinion; that's totally fine. In fact, I recommend you do so, as you'll have more peace of mind. I can help you get that second opinion and recommend other oncologists in the area with special expertise in your type of cancer. Just let me know if this is something you want to do."

Some patients would take me up on the offer, while others were content as is. I'd say over 90% did not seek a second opinion, but the other 10% did so for a variety of reasons. You read a few stories of various second opinions I encountered. An Australian study published in 2020 attempted to quantify the frequency of second opinions in oncology. Of over 350 patients surveyed, only 57 sought a second opinion, and their most common reason for doing so was their need for reassurance, followed by discussing treatment options. Among patients who did not seek a second opinion, the most common reason was their confidence and trust in the first doctor and opinion.

There are many reasons why patients seek another opinion. In my view, all of them are valid.

- **Confirmation of the diagnosis**: Not all diagnoses in oncology are straightforward, and some require special expertise. Patients and their families sometimes want assurance that the diagnosis is accurate and therefore the treatment is appropriate. For example, there are over 40 types of non-Hodgkin lymphomas and several types of acute myeloid leukemia, so knowing the correct diagnosis is essential. Usually, the second opinion physician needs to access the medical records and the pathology slides to perform a formal review and confirm the diagnosis. Occasionally, a new biopsy might be needed.

- **Confirmation of the best treatment**: For some cancers, there are several viable treatment choices, especially for the uncommon or rare ones. For others, the treatment choice is never in dispute. When a treatment is recommended, getting the same treatment recommendation from someone else provides patients with more confidence in the care they're receiving. Even though patients might be seeking the second opinion to discuss treatment options, the first step is always confirming the diagnosis. For some cancers, there can be more than one appropriate treatment choice, and the reason why one doctor recommends one choice versus another can be related to familiarity with the regimen or the doctor's perception of how a patient might tolerate the treatment. In other words, there can be more than one correct approach to the same disease, and patients want to discuss all the choices along with their pros and cons. This one is tough because it can lead to patients being confused, but with proper counseling, patients can understand why there are various choices or the lack of any viable choices.

- **Communication breakdown:** I cannot overstate how essential communication is. It's about having the medical care team available to patients. Is the doctor and their team available in an emergency? Do they return calls? Do they spend time discussing blood work and imaging studies? Are patients satisfied overall with the level of care received? This is a personal issue, but I have seen patients seeking another opinion after they have grown dissatisfied with how they are cared for. They might be receiving the correct therapy, but proper care is more than just delivering appropriate drugs. It's about caring for a patient as a whole. Only patients can answer the question on how well they're being treated. The cancer journey requires the right partner and the right hospital. How attentive to details is the medical team?

- **Clinical trials:** The next chapter focuses on clinical trials, but essentially these are programs by which some patients might be eligible for an experimental treatment that is not yet approved for their disease but is being studied at another clinic or institution. Getting another opinion about that and whether you qualify is sometimes a reason to go elsewhere. Your doctor likely knows whether you might be eligible and can call the larger center in the area inquiring on your behalf whether you may qualify for a clinical trial.

In a 2017 study, the range of second opinions in cancer patients varied widely, but in analyzing the data, researchers found that patients who had higher education sought second opinions more often. Patients' primary motivations were a perceived need for certainty or confirmation, a lack of trust, dissatisfaction with communication, and/or a need for more (personalized) information. Reported rates of diagnostic or therapeutic discrepancies between the first and second opinions ranged from 2% to 51% in the study.

If you have decided to seek a second opinion, here are the steps I suggest you take:

- Tell your oncologist that you want a second opinion. You'll need to trust me when I say this is very common and your oncologist will not be offended. In fact, if they get offended, you are probably better off with someone else anyway. Most oncologists will help you get the second opinion and even give you some insights on who to see and who not to see. How best to find the second opinion doctor can vary, but there are several avenues:
  ○ Your current oncologist might recommend who you should see.
  ○ Word of mouth—your friends and family members might know a good second opinion doctor.
  ○ Your insurance company might recommend several options.
  ○ Search the Find an Oncologist Database: https://www.cancer .net/find-cancer-doctor.
  ○ Search for the closest large academic center to you.

- Search the Medicare database: https://www.medicare.gov /care-compare/?providerType=Physician.
- Ask or research through patient advocacy groups.

- Check with your insurance company about the second opinion. Almost all insurance companies will pay for a second opinion if you have or suspect a cancer diagnosis. In fact, some insurance companies mandate the second opinion before agreeing to pay for the recommended therapy. While administrative staff at your oncologist's office can help you navigate the insurance maze, it never hurts for you to call your carrier and ask about costs and coverage.

- Have all your medical records ready. This might not be required in situations where the second opinion doctor has access to the electronic medical record system of your original oncologist. Some medical centers require that you send them the records ahead of time. I am no big fan of this as I have had my share of records lost through the mailing system, so if you mail your records, make sure you make copies and bring those with you to your second opinion visit. Medical records include progress notes from your doctor, imaging studies performed and their reports, laboratory data, and the pathology reports if you already had biopsies done.

Now that you have a second opinion visit secured, the same advice that I provided regarding your first visit applies here, with a few additional items:

- Don't go alone if you can; please bring a trusted friend or family member. You'll always need an extra set of ears to listen and take notes.

- Feel free to ask your doctor about recording the visit. If you ask, they won't be offended.

- Ask all the questions you had compiled ahead of the visit. Importantly, if there is a discrepancy between what the new doctor is recommending and what the first one suggested, ask so you understand why.

There is no question that getting a second opinion will make you feel more empowered and provide you with more confidence as you proceed on the treatment journey.

Take-Home Points

- Second opinions are always recommended.
- Don't be embarrassed asking for one.
- There are several databases to help you decide who to see as a second opinion, as well as your own oncologist's suggestions.
- Second opinions help in a variety of cases:
  - Confirm the diagnosis.
  - Confirm the optimal and ideal treatment.
  - Check the availability of clinical trials.
  - Improve communication and availability, and increase support staff.

CHAPTER 8

Clinical Trials

The science of today is the
technology of tomorrow.

—*Edward Teller*

ADVANCEMENTS IN SCIENCE have always been contingent
on asking questions and challenging the status quo. Let's face it,
someone a long time ago asked if the earth was flat, and here we are.
It's not.

Medicine has evolved over the years, and our knowledge of
how and when to treat patients has also progressed. As a society,
we owe these advances partly to clinical trials. Not uncommonly,
patients may be offered participation in clinical trials and are
asked to consider them. Over 90% of adult patients with cancer
decline participating in these studies; there are many reasons why,
but the most cited reason by patients and their families is that
these trials are experimental, and patients are not interested in
being a "guinea pig." Other reasons can be logistics, such as driving back and forth to the trial location; fear of side effects; the fact

that some patients might not get the new experimental drug that is hypothesized to be effective; and other requirements, such as frequent biopsies.

In fact, in a 2021 study, patients who were not enrolled in a clinical trial were surveyed to quantify their reasoning for not participating. The study found that the greatest patient-reported barriers were misperceptions about placebos, a desire to not feel like a human guinea pig, and uncertainty about efficacy of experimental therapies being studied in these trials.

I recall seeing a patient who had non-Hodgkin lymphoma that was not responding to the treatment his local oncologist had prescribed. Among other therapy options, I discussed with the patient and his daughter a clinical trial.

Daughter: So, will he get the drug?

CN: He might. The trial assigns half the enrolled patients participating to one drug and the other half to that same drug plus the new agent that we are exploring and that we just discussed.

Daughter: So, there are no guarantees that my dad will get that new drug?

CN: Correct. If he decides to participate in the trial, he may not receive the experimental new medication; he could be in the control group receiving the placebo. Please remember that we don't know how good that new drug is, and that is why the trial is being done. The computer assigns each patient to what treatment he or she would receive. I have no control over what your dad would get. We also don't know if the drug works . . .

My patient: I am not putting my health in the hands of a machine, and I don't see the benefit if you can't guarantee me getting that new drug. Thanks, but no thanks.

What Are Clinical Trials?

Simply put, clinical trials ask questions that physicians, researchers, and other healthcare professionals do not know the answers to but view as important for clinical care and potentially helpful in advancing science.

According to the National Institutes of Health (NIH), a clinical trial is defined as "a research study in which one or more human subjects are prospectively assigned to one or more interventions (which may include placebo or other control) to evaluate the effects of those interventions on health-related biomedical or behavioral outcomes." This definition might be too verbose, and by now you know that I like to simplify things. The best way to think of clinical trials is by understanding their scope and goals.

Phase 1 Clinical Trials

Phase 1 studies often test new drugs that are given to people for the first time. Essentially, researchers are asking whether the treatment is safe to be given to humans and what the highest dose that we could administer safely is. Of course, since we don't know if the drug being studied works in humans, patients who are enrolled in these studies must have exhausted all known treatments that could work for them. Prior to initiating a phase 1 study on a drug, the drug itself would have been tested in animals and in the laboratory to demonstrate at least that it is appropriate to give to humans. However, the proper dose is usually unknown, and the side effects are not well characterized. Simply, these phase 1 studies help decide the best way to administer therapy, what cancer type it might help treat, and whether it is safe to continue studying it.

In general, the first patients enrolled in a phase 1 clinical trial get a low dose of the experimental drug. If side effects are viewed as tolerable, then more patients are allowed to be on that trial, but often they receive a higher dose than the original ones. The doses are increased gradually as more patients are entered in the study until patients encounter side effects that are considered not tolerable or unacceptable based on the physicians' judgment. So, really, the main concern here is safety, but at the same time, knowing the proper dose that patients can receive with reasonable expected toxicity allows further study of the drug.

This approach might be viewed by some as unacceptable and a far cry from science. How could we keep increasing a dose of a drug until patients can no longer tolerate it? Opponents of this approach have argued that we need to study various genes in each patient, which can help us determine whether they can tolerate a drug and whether they might respond to that drug. This evolving field is now called *pharmacogenomics.*

Importantly, physicians should explain to patients that the main purpose of phase 1 studies is not to know whether the drugs being studied work but rather to better understand their dosing in humans and the possible toxicities. This does not mean that patients would never benefit from phase 1 trials, as some of them for sure do. I would imagine, however, that telling a patient that the sole purpose of being enrolled in a phase 1 study is to find the proper dose for future trials is not always going to go well. But patients could certainly benefit from being in these trials. The majority of cancer drugs were in a phase 1 study at some point.

In December 2000, I was attending the annual meeting of the American Society of Hematology (ASH) in San Francisco. During the plenary session, top scientific presentations are discussed and shared with thousands of people anticipating results and data. Dr. Brian Druker from Oregon University presented results of a phase 1 study using a drug called at the time STI-571 (subsequently, it was named imatinib [Gleevec]) in patients with a form of leukemia called chronic myeloid leukemia. The drug had minimal side effects, which was reassuring, but what was striking were the efficacy results. The drug worked in most patients, even though the trial was not designed to explore how effective it was.

I was an oncology fellow at the time, and I recall sitting by one of my colleagues who was also doing his fellowship at Northwestern University. I looked at him as one slide was being projected after another.

"Is this for real?" I asked.

He was silent, absorbing the data. I continued in a hushed voice so that the thousands in the plenary session hallway didn't hear me. "I actually did a bone marrow biopsy on a couple of patients who were on this trial," I elaborated with a proud tone.

The drug and its data made it to the *Time* magazine cover; arguably, imatinib and subsequent similar drugs that treat this disease have forever revolutionized the way cancer is viewed and treated.

One of the salient points to remember about phase 1 studies is that in some of them, patients with different types of cancers can be enrolled. Also, phase 1 trials do not have a placebo, and the patient will always receive the drug that is being studied. Generally, these studies are not large, and often only a few dozen patients are included.

Phase 2 Clinical Trials

Once a drug is determined as safe and we know how best to administer it to patients, we must understand how good it is. Phase 2 studies are designed to investigate the efficacy of a drug in a specific type of cancer. Generally, patients do not get a placebo, and they all receive the drug being studied. There are scenarios in which phase 2 studies also explore the best way to give a drug (IV or pills, etc.) and could assign patients to one route versus another.

Deciding which type of cancer to study a drug in is often based on the researcher's views of the published scientific investigations that help determine whether the mechanism of action for that drug might help patients with that specific type of cancer. Moreover, information gathered from phase 1 studies can direct researchers to determine which cancers should be targeted in phase 2 trials.

Phase 2 trials are still small and enroll anywhere from 20–100 patients, although some of them can be larger. Often the dose and frequency of the drug given are based on what was found during phase 1 studies. To determine whether the drug works, patients who receive the therapy are monitored closely and undergo serial imaging studies to measure the tumors and determine whether they are shrinking.

Depending on how much of the tumor shrinks, physicians determine whether the cancer has fully, partially, or never responded to treatment. Some tumors do not grow or shrink and remain stable; that might still be valuable for some patients.

It is very important to set the expectations properly and explain to patients and their families the goal of treatment.

I saw a patient with metastatic prostate cancer that had spread to the bones and the lymph glands. The patient was referred for a clinical trial that was available at the University of Chicago. It was a phase 2 study looking at an oral drug designed to stop the growth of the cancer.

Patient: Will the cancer go away?

CN: Our goal is to control the cancer. Your cancer is in the "controllable" stage, and we cannot cure it, but we are hoping to make things better.

Patient: What should I expect?

CN: My hope is that some of these lymph glands shrink and maybe some of the bone disease gets better. I will also be monitoring your serum PSA levels to assess if you're responding.

Patient: What if nothing shrinks?

CN: If nothing shrinks and nothing grows, that is also good. Look, having a cancer that remains stable is still a good achievement if you maintain your active lifestyle and quality of life. We need to keep it at bay, even if it doesn't shrink.

No shrinkage and no growth are what oncologists have historically called *stable disease*; the disease is still there but is stable. This is not a bad outcome as long as the patient is not having detrimental symptoms or side effects. If patients encounter long periods of time without the cancer getting bigger, it is an important achievement in terms of incurable conditions.

I would argue that it is very important to look at quality of life anytime we conduct these studies. Shrinkage of tumors at arbitrary percentages might not always translate into patients feeling better. Many researchers have advocated that incorporating quality-of-life assessments is a critical component of all studies.

If phase 2 studies suggest a drug is effective in a particular cancer, researchers might consider a large phase 3 study to investigate whether it should replace current standard therapy for that particular cancer.

Phase 3 Clinical Trials

Simply put, phase 3 trials ask the question: "Are these new therapies better than what we are currently using for that specific cancer?" Most of these trials enroll a large number of patients measured in hundreds. There are times when placebo is used in phase 3 trials, but rarely alone. The results of phase 2 studies must be impressive enough to propose that a new drug or regimen can change the standard of care being used by healthcare professionals.

Consider the example of how treating a form of non-Hodgkin lymphoma changed forever in the early 2000s. Historically, diffuse large B-cell lymphoma, the most common form of non-Hodgkin lymphoma, had been treated with a cocktail of chemotherapy drugs (we call the regimen CHOP).

In the early 2000s, European investigators hypothesized that adding a drug called rituximab to CHOP might improve outcomes. This was based on preliminary phase 2 studies that showed excellent efficacy when rituximab was used with CHOP.

At another ASH plenary session I attended, Bertrand Coiffier from France shared with the world how adding rituximab to CHOP improved overall survival of patients with this aggressive form of non-Hodgkin lymphoma. Within months, the new regimen, the so-called R-CHOP, replaced CHOP and became the new standard based on that European phase 3 trial.

Sometimes, in these phase 3 trials, the physician and the patient are aware of what the patient is receiving, but there are trials where neither is aware. The latter form is called a *double-blind trial.*

Phase 3 trials try to replace the current standard based on showing that a new regimen is better than or as good as the current therapy but is less toxic. Recently, and due to increasing costs of cancer care, some studies have started incorporating cost of drugs and health care as part of these studies with the idea that if two regimens are equally effective and equally toxic, maybe we should adopt the one that is less expensive.

One of the salient features of phase 3 studies, and one that I have personally criticized, is the strict inclusion and exclusion criteria. These are essentially a checklist of characteristics that enrolled patients must possess to be in that study. My criticism is that these criteria often overlook the characteristics of patients seen in routine clinical care, or what has been labeled as "real-world."

In 2019, I was invited to give a lecture on real-world evidence as part of a healthcare disparities conference sponsored by the Binaytara

Foundation, a nonprofit foundation that aims to mitigate disparities in cancer care globally.

As I took the podium, I asked the audience, "How many of you are involved in clinical trials?"

Many hands were raised among the 100-plus attendees in this medium-sized conference room.

I continued, "How often did you want to enroll a patient in a clinical trial but found that your patient's hemoglobin was 8, while the trial mandated a hemoglobin of 9?"

Few hands remained raised.

I continued to my punch line: "Now, be honest; how many ended up transfusing your patient with one or two units of blood to increase the hemoglobin value above that threshold so that you could enroll your patient?"

A few brave hands remained up.

I was alluding to the fact that inclusion and exclusion criteria can be strict. Some of these criteria are based on solid scientific grounds, but many are not. They are designed to enroll patients who are fit and relatively healthy, despite their cancers, so that they have the highest chance of benefiting from the trial. I was also hinting at how physicians sometimes try to work around this impractical "strictness" when they view it as unnecessary. In the scenario I provided, physicians would give blood to patients to raise their hemoglobin enough to allow enrollment in the clinical trial.

My argument has always been that we need to make inclusion/exclusion criteria as close as possible to the characteristics of patients seen in the real world. This is the only way to ensure that the results of these studies are transferable to all patients across the spectrum. This idea, called *pragmatism*, has now become popular. Designing pragmatic clinical trials has become the best approach, and in fact, regulatory bodies (agencies that eventually decide whether a drug gets approved and can be sold) have now incentivized manufacturers to ensure pragmatism in their studies—that they enroll patients who represent real-world demographics and characteristics.

Phase 4 Clinical Trials

After a drug or a regimen is approved and being used by physicians to treat patients for a particular indication, the reality is that we don't know if it works in all patients with that indication. From a purely scientific standpoint, we can only say that it works in patients who have inclusion/exclusion criteria similar to those of the patients who were in the drug's clinical trial.

Phase 4 clinical trials were incepted to monitor drugs approved by the Food and Drug Administration (FDA) over a long period of time and to monitor how these drugs perform in thousands of patients, especially those who differ from the original patients studied (such as minorities, older adults, or patients who have other medical problems). Phase 4 allows us to look at practical aspects, such as adherence to therapy, cost of treatment, and long-term safety, among others.

The Institutional Review Board (IRB)

Clinical trials are highly regulated to ensure that patients are served right and are protected. To ensure the trial is sound and patient rights are preserved, every trial is reviewed by a committee composed of individuals of varying backgrounds and scientific abilities. This committee is called the *institutional review board*, or the IRB.

I was fortunate to serve on an IRB for two years. We met every two weeks to review various clinical trials, not just oncology trials. Our role was to provide an independent review of the research studies to ensure that the conduct was ethical and that the trials adhered to federal regulations, state laws, and other requirements. On the IRB I served on, there was an ethicist, a nurse, several physicians of different specialties, patient advocates, pharmacists, and pastoral services, among other disciplines. When we conferred, we discussed the trial, ensured that it was ethical, and often asked the trial investigator to present to us a synopsis of his or her theory. We then voted on what should be done. Sometimes, we raised questions that the researchers needed to address before we approved it.

The IRB began in 1974 when the National Research Act was signed into law. The act created the National Commission for the Protection of Human Subjects of Biomedical and Behavioral Research. This commission was charged with identifying the basic ethical principles that underlie the conduct of biomedical and behavioral research and to develop guidelines for research involving human subjects. Research can raise ethical questions, such as the reported abuses of human subjects during World War II and the US Tuskegee syphilis trial in which rural Black men with syphilis were not told they were participating in research and were subsequently denied treatment for their disease when penicillin became a known cure.

The Nuremberg Code, created in 1947, was drafted as a result of the Nuremberg war crimes trials of Nazi physicians and scientists who had conducted atrocious biomedical experimentation on concentration camp prisoners. The code is composed of certain basic principles that must be observed to satisfy the moral, ethical, and legal requirements for conducting human research, and it has become the prototype of many later codes. Another set of guidelines is the Declaration of Helsinki drafted in 1964, which allows for humans with diminished capacity to participate in research if consent is obtained from their legal guardian.

When discussing ethics, it is important to define what the IRB looks at and reviews. This is outlined in what is called the *Belmont Report*, which summarizes the ethical principles to use:

- Respect for persons: to protect the autonomy and privacy rights of participants
- Beneficence: do no harm and make the most of benefits while reducing risks
- Justice

I was never paid for my services on the local IRB that I served on. IRB members generally volunteer their services to review these clinical trials and ensure human protection.

Despite these regulations and safeguards, many patients and their families remain concerned that these trials will treat them like "guinea pigs." Explaining these details to patients being considered for clinical trials is essential. It removes one barrier, but certainly not all barriers, to increased enrollment.

One of the most critical parts of IRB roles is to review the "informed consent," the document that patients read, review, and sign. This document must outline the purpose of the study and what patients should expect. Importantly, it must be written in very simple language that a student in elementary school could read and comprehend.

I always taught my students not to exaggerate expected benefits and downplay potential toxicities of a trial drug when discussing with a patient. It's not unusual to see that. I recall watching one of my hematology fellows consenting a patient to be enrolled in a trial.

Fellow: This study looks at this drug that we think is very effective. Side effects are minimal. Nothing that we can't control.

Patient: So, it's going to work.

Fellow: Most likely it will; it is a great option for you.

Afterward, I spoke with my fellow about how she consented the patient. Using the phrase "great option" is exaggerating. Stating "very effective" is likely inappropriate. We really don't know that the drug is effective to start with, so we can't propose that it can be very effective. She graciously accepted the teaching points, and we went back to spend more time with the patient reasonably discussing the study.

Clinical trials are important for advancing science, and patients who are enrolled might benefit from these studies. My hope is that you recognize that there are so many safeguards to protect your rights and participation and that you would discuss the proposed trials with your doctor seriously, without dismissing them outright.

Take-Home Points

- Clinical trials are recommended for all cancers.
- Researchers are working on mitigating the barriers to be enrolled in trials by making them more applicable to patients seen in the real world and by having less restricted inclusion/exclusion criteria.
- There are four different phases to clinical trials.
- The institutional review board (IRB) is a committee that reviews all clinical trials to ensure human subject protection and ethical conduct of these studies.

CHAPTER 9

Treating the Cancer: Surgery

*What we know is a drop,
what we don't know is an ocean.*

—*Isaac Newton*

HE WAS WEAK and fatigued as he walked into my exam room, accompanied by his family. A week prior, he was diagnosed with lymphoma after lymph nodes appeared on the left side of his neck. As we got to the point of discussing treatment, he asked, "Are we going to take these nodes out?" Knowing that most patients might have already researched a bit about their disease, I had assumed that he would have known that we don't treat lymphomas with surgery. Many patients need confirmation of their own research findings and a more elaborate explanation.

"Lymphomas are not treated with surgery," I replied, "although we need surgery to diagnose it, just like what happened to you last week when they removed the lymph node from your neck."

"Why didn't they remove all the nodes and call it a day?" he asked.

"Because even if they did, it doesn't mean that there is no cancer left. This cancer is not treated with surgery but rather with other types of treatments. Not all cancers are treated by removing the tumors. Surgery is not the answer for all cancers."

Another patient I saw was referred because of a growth on her colon. I explained that surgery is the cornerstone of treatment, but sometimes we give additional therapy after the tumor is removed. I emphasized that the only way to cure this cancer is to indeed remove it surgically and then decide what the next steps are.

"Your tumor is localized; it has not spread—it is in the curative stage," I said. "Once it is removed, we will have more information as to whether you need something more."

I recall another patient who had lung cancer that was removed surgically followed by several rounds of chemotherapy to reduce the risk of his cancer coming back (see chapter 10 on chemotherapy). Two years after he completed the chemotherapy, his cancer unfortunately returned as a growth on his adrenal gland. When I saw him to decide on next steps, I advised that we had to do a PET scan to evaluate whether any cancer had spread elsewhere besides the adrenal gland. Sure enough, the PET scan showed no cancer spread except in the adrenal gland. His brain MRI was also negative. We ended up doing a biopsy of the adrenal gland to know exactly what we were dealing with. The results came back consistent with the same cancer that he had a couple of years back.

"This is good news," I said. "I recommend that you see the surgeon and we work on removing the adrenal gland as there is no cancer anywhere else."

"You had told me before that if the cancer spreads, then we don't do surgery and we can't cure it," he reminded me. "I believe this is why we did chemotherapy originally after surgery, so it doesn't come back."

"I understand," I responded empathetically. "I am very sorry that it did, but it is good news that it came back to only one location and one location only. We still have a chance to cure this cancer, and we can do so by removing the adrenal gland."

Every cancer situation is different and nuanced. Some cancers are only treated with surgery while others are never treated surgically. Some cancers that spread are still treated with surgery, while others are never approached with a knife. Deciding on how we treat each cancer requires knowing the biology of the cancer being treated, patient-specific conditions, and goals of care, which are goals specific to each patient.

When it comes to surgery for cancers, it's important to recognize that there are different goals of performing surgery and different types of surgical techniques that can be performed.

Goals of Cancer Surgery

- **Diagnosis**: Some tumors are not easily accessible to get a biopsy. Recall that the only way to diagnose cancer is by removing a piece of tissue and examining it under the microscope. If the tumors are internal, we have no choice but to do a surgical procedure to get access to that internal area. If that is the only area where there is an abnormal growth, the surgeon might elect to remove the entire growth at the same time of doing the internal biopsy. Bottom line, we sometimes need to do surgery to simply know the type of cancer we are dealing with. I call this a diagnostic surgery based on its goal.

- **Removing the tumor**: There are many reasons to remove the tumor.
  - *Curative surgery*: This is a scenario where we know that the tumor has not spread to distant organs, and by removing it completely, we increase the chances of cure. Oftentimes, the tumor is removed plus some healthy surrounding tissues to ensure that every part of the tumor has been excised. What is important in most of these surgeries is removing the surrounding lymph glands. Doing so helps determine the stage

of the cancer. As we discussed, it is so important to know the stage (curable or controllable), and we cannot do so in most instances without removing the lymph glands surrounding the cancer growth. This is because most cancers spread by going to the closest lymph nodes, so by resecting these, we can tell if the cancer has started going elsewhere. In some cancers, taking more nodes is better because if we don't take enough nodes, the remaining ones might be involved, and we just wouldn't know. The correct stage determines whether patients need more treatment after surgery (such as chemotherapy and/or radiation). Therefore, having these surgeries performed by a surgeon who understands these nuances is critical for optimal results.

o *Curative surgery of a spread*: The reasoning behind this is similar to the case of my patient who had a growth on his adrenal gland. Some cancers recur in only one location, and in certain circumstances removing that sole recurring growth could provide the patient with a cure. Some cancers at the time of their initial diagnosis could be found in one other location amenable to removal, and on occasion, the original tumor as well as that solo spread are both removed. There are several examples similar to the case of my adrenal gland patient. I'll never forget my patient who had colon cancer that returned only to a small area in the liver. After removing that solitary liver lesion, he lived for 10 more years and died from natural causes without relapse.

o *Debulking surgery*: Sometimes, removing most of the tumor even when we cannot remove it completely is better than no removal at all. One cancer that comes to mind here involves the brain and is called glioblastoma multiforme, or GBM. Because of its location and sometimes size, occasionally the growth cannot be entirely removed. However, removing most of it is certainly better than nothing at all because doing so makes patients live longer, especially if they receive additional treatment afterward, such as chemotherapy and/or radiation. Another example is ovarian cancer, where removing much of the tumors helps improve patients' outcomes.

○ *Palliative surgery*: This is the type of surgery that we know will not cure the cancer and may not help patients live longer, but we still do it because it will make patients feel better. It might relieve some of their symptoms and lead to a better quality of life. I'll never forget one of my dearest patients who was diagnosed with pancreatic cancer. The growth on the pancreas was large enough that it blocked parts of his intestines, and it affected his ability to eat. The cancer had spread to his liver and was not curable, but after speaking with him and consulting with the surgeon, we decided on surgery to bypass the blockage, which would help him not vomit every time he ate. My patient tolerated the surgery well and was able to receive chemotherapy afterward. He had a good quality of life for the subsequent 11 months he lived. We all knew that this bypass surgery would not cure him, but it still helped him tremendously.

I had a patient with multiple myeloma, a cancer of the bone marrow that also makes the skeletal bones fragile and prone to breaking. He had severe back pain due to an almost broken vertebra. He underwent a spinal surgery to stabilize the bones and prevent fractures in that area that could have damaged the spinal cord. This was "supportive and palliative surgery" but not the mainstay treatment of his disease.

• **Other kinds of surgery**

○ *Reconstructive surgery*: This is commonly done to repair or replace damaged or missing tissue. An example of such surgery is breast reconstruction surgery for women with breast cancer after a mastectomy. Often, a plastic surgeon is involved, and reconstruction can involve breast implants, but occasionally a woman's own tissue can be used after mastectomy. Not every patient chooses to undergo reconstruction surgery as this is an elective procedure, but in my opinion, consulting with a physician about the options is important so that the patient makes an informed decision on whether this is the proper approach. There are many other examples where reconstructive surgery might be considered, such as repairing defects in the head and neck area that is affected by cancer or skin grafts after extensive melanoma surgery. In general, timing and technique for all these vary, and they are beyond the scope of this book.

○ *Preventive surgery*: There are situations when the doctor recommends surgery to prevent cancer from developing in organs if left unresected. Essentially, this is a risk-reducing procedure that decreases a person's high-risk predisposition to cancer. This is often done in patients who carry a particular genetic mutation known to increase the risk of developing cancer significantly. An example is a mutation in a gene called *BRCA-1*, which increases the risk of developing breast and ovarian cancers. Sometimes, removing both breasts is recommended, and doing so reduces the risk of developing breast cancer by over 90%. Occasionally, removing both ovaries in women with *BRCA-1* is also recommended. So, when the risk of developing cancer in a particular organ is very high, removing it surgically might be recommended. In these scenarios, I always recommend a discussion with a genetic counselor as well as a psychologist. These are not easy recommendations or decisions, as we are recommending resection of healthy organs in someone who does not have cancer because we have scientific reasons that the risk of developing the cancer in the future is very high. You can imagine how difficult this decision can be.

Types of Cancer Surgery

- **Open surgery**: Its name explains what gets done. The surgeon makes a large cut and removes the tumor and surrounding tissue where applicable. This is done under general anesthesia.

- **Minimally invasive surgery**: As the name implies, there are no large cuts here. The surgeon makes few small cuts and inserts a thin tube attached to a camera in one of them. That tube is called a laparoscope, and the surgery is called "laparoscopic surgery." The surgeon can see the images projected from the camera on a monitor, which improves visualization of the inner organs. Surgeons who have perfected this technique cite published peer-reviewed literature showing that this approach helps patients recover faster with minimal scars and shorter hospital stays, leading to better outcomes.

- **Robotic-assisted surgery**: This advanced form of minimally invasive surgery offers better visualization of the operative field and helps the surgeon better control the surgical instruments. The most commonly used robotic surgical system includes a camera arm and mechanical arms attached to surgical instruments. The surgeon controls these arms while sitting near the operating field.

- **Cryosurgery or cryotherapy**: This is like freezing the cancer. Extreme cold is produced by liquid nitrogen or argon gas to destroy the cancer. When done on external cancers like skin cancer, the doctor can apply the liquid nitrogen directly on the abnormal area. For internal organs, a device is used to enter the body through a very small skin cut, and the gas is applied directly on the internal tumor. Imaging is used to more precisely apply the gas. The body absorbs these dying tumors eventually. Proponents of this technology argue that it causes much less pain and complications than standard surgery, but not every patient is indeed a candidate for cryosurgery as this technique depends on the actual cancer, location, and whether the cryo procedure is being done as a replacement to regular surgery because the patient cannot tolerate the standard procedure. For some patients who undergo cryosurgery, no hospital stay is needed as many of these surgeries can be done with local anesthesia. One of the attractions of cryosurgery is that it can be done when tumors cannot be removed using regular surgical techniques or when the cancer stops responding to usual therapies. The biggest drawback to cryosurgery in my opinion is that there are little data to assure patients that undergoing this procedure cures cancers or prolongs survival.

- **Laser surgery**: Lasers are beams of light used to destroy cancer cells or those cells at highest risk of becoming cancerous. This surgery can also serve as a local treatment to a specific area in the body where the tumor is located. As an oncologist, I relied on my consultants to decide whether this type of therapy was doable and reasonable. When treating superficial cancers, carbon dioxide or argon lasers are used, but when treating internal organs, a material called yttrium-aluminum-garnet is used.

- **Hyperthermia**: During hyperthermia, areas of interest are exposed to very high temperatures, as high as 113°F, which will kill the cancer cells. Doctors use imaging studies to introduce probes with tiny thermometers, but how hyperthermia is introduced to the tumors depends on their location (external accessible or internal organs). The term "radiofrequency ablation" is used when doctors introduce radio waves to heat and kill cancer cells by inserting probes or needles into the tumor. An example is when heated chemotherapy is internalized into the peritoneal cavity (the space within the abdomen that contains the intestines, liver, and stomach), usually during surgery with general anesthesia. Treatment with hyperthermia requires very experienced surgeons and medical centers. The scientist in me remains skeptical as to whether this approach indeed makes patients live longer. The research findings have been mixed. Side effects include pain, swelling, and burns in various organs.

Risks of Surgery

How doctors frame risks versus benefits of any medical procedure is important in how patients interpret the information. Many years ago, I read an example in *Thinking, Fast and Slow*, a book written by Dr. Daniel Kahneman, which illustrates the concept.

Consider a surgeon who tells a patient that their risk of making a full recovery with a surgical intervention is 90%. This sounds great. The same doctor tells another patient that the risk of the surgery not working is 10%; to the second patient, this sounds awful because that risk feels high, even if the truth is that the surgery works 90% of the time. It's how we convey the information that matters. Communication is key, and it is why I dedicate an entire chapter to the topic later in the book.

There is no surgical procedure that carries zero risk. There is always a risk, but the percentage of risk varies based on the procedure, the cancer, the surgeon's skills and expertise, and the patient's condition. Common problems from surgery are pain and infection. Other complications can include cardiac events and pulmonary complications or blood clots. It is why some doctors ask a cardiologist to see the patient pre-op to ensure that the risks are acceptable. A cardiologist might sometimes order a stress test before surgery to make sure that the patient's heart can withstand the operation. To prevent clots, the doctor will place patients on blood thinners that often start before the operation takes place; this regimen can continue for days or weeks after surgery is complete, depending on the type of surgery and the potential perceived risk of developing these clots. In a cancer situation, incomplete surgery—the inability to remove the entire tumor when this was the goal—is another problem that can lead to downstream effects in terms of management. In certain situations, patients might not be able to start eating soon after surgery, and the medical team might elect to start nutritional supplementation by the vein or another route. Another surgical risk is loss of organ function due to the actual operation. Say that the bladder or a kidney needs to be removed. Removing an organ leads to loss of its function, but there are ways to compensate for these lost functions when needed.

All these examples illustrate that there are risks simply because of surgery (any kind of surgery) and risks based on the type of tumor and condition of the cancer that is being operated on.

Be Armed with Questions

I always make a point to tell patients, "No question is stupid." Toward the end of my consultations with patients and throughout the visits, I always emphasize that they can ask questions and that no question is ever unacceptable. You'd be surprised to know how uncomfortable some patients are in asking questions, and maybe this is partly the fault of some doctors who are perceived as unapproachable. But this is your body, your life, and your battle. It is important to ask all the questions and not be embarrassed to ask them and demand answers. If the doctor is uncomfortable answering these basic questions, my advice is to seek another opinion. Here is a list of suggested questions to ask; while not inclusive, these are a good start:

- Why am I having this surgery?
- Is this surgery going to cure my cancer on its own?

- How much normal tissue will be removed?
- Do I need more tests before we go to surgery? Will we do tests after surgery to ensure its success?
- Are there other surgical options available to me?
- Is surgery the only choice to move forward?
- How long will the operation last?
- Will I need general anesthesia?
- Will you do the surgery? Or is there a team of surgeons that will work with you?
- Do I need other treatments after I recover from surgery?
- How long do you think my recovery will take?
- Is there anything I can do to expedite my recovery?
- How many similar surgeries have you performed?
- How long do I need to stay in the hospital before I go home?
- What are the major complications that I should anticipate?
- How likely am I to experience any or all of these complications?
- What can I do or what should I not do to minimize the risks of these complications?
- How long will it take until I get the pathology results of the removed tumor?
- Do you think you can remove the entire tumor?
- If I experience side effects after I go home, how can I reach you?
- If you're not available, who can I contact?
- Can your office check on my financial responsibility and whether my insurance covers this surgery?
- Does my insurance cover the anesthesia team that will take care of me?

- Will I need rehab after surgery? If so, inpatient or outpatient rehab?

- Can I return to work or school after surgery? How soon after? Can I return full time?

If you do not understand an answer to a question, say so. Take notes or have someone with you to take notes. Ask every question that concerns you. You would do the same if you were buying a car, so now is not the time to be shy.

Take-Home Points

- Not all cancers are treated with surgery, but many are.

- There are various reasons to perform surgery on a cancer.

- There are different techniques to perform cancer surgeries.

- No surgical intervention is without some kind of risk. Please ask questions to understand the risks versus benefits, indication, and potential alternatives.

- Some patients might require additional therapy after undergoing surgery to further treat the cancer, while others might undergo treatment (in the form of chemotherapy or radiation) before having surgery.

CHAPTER 10

Treating the Cancer:
Chemotherapy

Never bend your head.
Always hold it high.
Look the world straight in the eye.

—*Helen Keller*

MY PATIENT WAS CLEARLY CONFUSED. His eyes and body
language implied perplexity; somehow coming to a cancer clinic was
more stressful and problematic to him than the surgery he'd had a few
weeks ago. His loving wife appeared equally puzzled. It wasn't unusual for me to ask my first-time patients if they knew why they were
referred. It always gave me a sense of their understanding of the disease and their overall knowledge.

"I am not sure why they wanted me to see you," he protested.
"My surgeon told me that they took everything out. Everything," he
emphasized.

"She did take everything out," I replied.

"Great. So, why am I here? The cancer is out. She said something about needing chemotherapy, and I don't get why I need it if she took everything out."

"Your surgeon is excellent. She and her team took everything they could see out. Indeed, they did. But they cannot take out things they cannot see."

I could sense that his confusion increased. "Look," I said, "surgeons will remove everything they can possibly see and then some. They even remove healthy tissue that surrounds the tumor, and they remove some lymph nodes that are close by, but in the end they can only remove what they find and see. By examining the tissues under the microscope, however, we can determine how high the risk of the cancer coming back is; the additional treatment that we give after surgery is to minimize that risk of recurrence."

Despite removing everything visible during surgery, there is an inherent risk that some cells will be left behind because the surgeon cannot see these cells to remove them. We call these cells "micrometastases," and their risk of being present after surgery varies based on what the pathologist finds. If the risk is high enough, patients might receive additional treatment after surgery. If the risk is very minimal, no more treatment is usually given following surgery.

"So," my patient continued, "what you're telling me is that the surgeon took it all out, but she took what she saw, and there may be cells left behind that we need to kill with your treatment."

"Exactly," I said. "The chemotherapy you will receive will hopefully kill these invisible cells, and it prevents them from growing back and causing a recurrence. At the least, it minimizes the risk of recurrence, but it may not eliminate it completely. From looking at the tumor that was removed, the benefits of giving you treatment to eradicate these cells appears to outweigh the potential risks."

Satisfied with my answer, we moved on to discuss the type of chemotherapy he would receive and how we would manage its side effects.

I recall seeing a patient who had esophageal cancer; he was having difficulty swallowing and had lost a substantial amount of weight. The surgeon did not feel that he could do surgery right away, and at the time some studies were suggesting that giving chemotherapy before surgery could help patients achieve better surgical outcomes and potentially make them live longer.

"Giving chemotherapy before surgery will hopefully shrink the tumor and get you to eat, gain weight, and be more ready for surgery," I explained. "The surgeon can likely do a better job with a smaller tumor."

"I understand," he responded.

"It also allows us to see firsthand how sensitive your cancer is to the chemotherapy drugs. Seeing shrinkage means your cells are sensitive to the therapy. If we don't see shrinkage, we might need to switch treatment or proceed with surgery sooner rather than later."

My patient had an excellent outcome. He underwent surgery and then underwent additional treatment with chemotherapy.

In oncology, we refer to giving chemotherapy after the surgery or after the definitive local cancer treatment is complete as adjuvant therapy, and we call giving chemotherapy before surgery neo-adjuvant therapy. The first patient I mentioned was to undergo adjuvant therapy, while my second patient underwent neoadjuvant chemotherapy.

In some cancers, surgery is never needed, and chemotherapy is the only needed therapy to cure the cancer. There are occasions, however, where chemotherapy is used to control the cancer and improve symptoms. The latter scenario is what we usually call "palliative chemotherapy," and the former is defined as "definitive or curative" chemotherapy.

What Is Chemotherapy?

As the name implies, chemotherapy uses chemicals that are supposed to stop cancer cells from growing and kill them where they are. Every cell in our body goes through "the cycle of life" in order to divide and multiply. Cancer cells do so as well, except much faster than normal cells. Chemotherapy drugs attack cancer cells at various stages of the cell cycle. These drugs are poisons, but they are supposed to poison the cancer cells and inhibit their ability to multiply by damaging their DNA. Sometimes, however, these drugs affect the noncancerous cells, which is why patients can experience side effects. How chemotherapy does that varies based on the type of chemotherapy drug, and therefore, chemotherapy agents are categorized based on their mechanism of action.

Patients fear chemotherapy, as these drugs can cause many side effects. Some fear it to a degree that they forgo such treatment because they think that the chemotherapy is worse than the cancer itself. It's normal to fear taking poison! But these toxic chemicals are carefully tested to do the least amount of damage with the most amount of effect. I have often started discussing chemotherapy drugs with my patients by telling them that these drugs are not the weapons of mass destruction they hear about on TV. So, what are the types of chemotherapy out there?

Chemotherapy drugs generally work better on cells that are rapidly multiplying. Cancer cells are usually growing and dividing much faster than normal cells, and therefore, chemotherapy can affect cancer cells more than normal cells. That is the primary goal of this treatment approach: to contain and cancel the rapid cancer cell growth.

Alkylating Agents

Some argue that alkylating agents are the oldest type of chemotherapy. They are originally derived from mustard gas, which was first used as a chemical weapon in World War I and other armed conflicts. Compounds belonging to this family prevent cell growth by damaging its DNA, leading to cell death (what we called apoptosis in a prior chapter). Sometimes, if cell death does not ensue, damaged DNA of the healthy cells can lead to future development of other cancers.

These compounds are called alkylating agents because they can alkylate (they add one or more alkyl groups to a compound in a chemical way to produce another compound) anything in the cell—DNA, RNA, and proteins. What's important to recognize is that these compounds bind to the DNA and exert their anticancer effects. The fraction of the cells that die from these agents is directly related to the dose of the drug being administered. There are too many chemotherapy names that belong to this class to list here, and you don't need to remember these names, but you do need to write on a piece of paper the name of the chemotherapy drugs your doctor prescribes.

Often, I would be asked by a patient and their family members how a chemotherapy drug works. The simplest answer has always been, "They interfere with how cancer cells grow and multiply and prevent that from happening; they affect DNA in the cancer cells, so they stop dividing." They can affect normal cells too, and this leads to side effects that we need to manage. I try not to go into too much of the science of the drugs, but if you find you'd like to know more about them and the particular drugs you will take for your cancer, your oncologist should be able to give you more detail. Don't be afraid to ask.

Antimetabolites

As the name implies, antimetabolites are chemicals that prevent the use of a "metabolite," a compound that evolves from normal metabolism. They can have similar structure to the metabolite they're inhibiting. This process in turn leads to preventing and stopping cell growth and to slowing the cancer cells from continuing to multiply. Antimetabolites interfere with DNA and RNA synthesis, which impairs cancer cells' proliferation. These drugs exert their effect by either blocking the enzymes required for DNA synthesis or becoming incorporated into the DNA or RNA.

Antitumor Antibiotics

The name "antitumor antibiotics" is deceiving as these are not real antibiotics that patients take for an infection. This class of drugs interrupts cell division and multiplication by preventing the formation of the RNA from the DNA.

Topoisomerase Inhibitors

Topoisomerases are enzymes that alter how the DNA coils on each other. There are two such enzymes, and they are essential to the DNA function that eventually leads to transcription, as we discussed in chapter 1. Some chemotherapy drugs inhibit these enzymes, thereby preventing cell growth and eventually cell death.

It's challenging to cover every chemotherapy drug, every category, and every mechanism, but the descriptions I have provided illustrate the general principles of how these drugs operate.

How Do We Give Chemotherapy?

Chemotherapy can be given to any patient through various routes.

- **Intravenously**: Basically, the chemotherapy drugs are infused through tubes connected to a needle that is inserted in the vein. Sometimes these needles are taken out after the infusion is complete, but at times we insert a device that makes infusing the chemotherapy easier and possibly less damaging to the veins.

That device is called a "port-a-cath" and is used to draw blood as well as to give chemotherapy, blood transfusion, or any other infusion. The port looks like a bump under the skin; it is most often placed on the right side of the chest, and it can be accessed by a needle. That bump is attached to a catheter that is guided into a large vein above the right side of the heart. Sometimes we keep that port throughout treatment and remove it once therapy is completed. I have had patients who felt uncomfortable removing the port even after treatment was done, voicing concerns that taking the port out might make the cancer return. But removing the device is likely better than keeping it in. I have always relied on the amazing nurses I worked with to decide whether a patient needed that device. Their recommendations were based on whether the chemotherapy being administered could damage the vein and leak outside of the veins into the tissues (the medical terminology is "vesicant chemo"), whether the patient was considered a hard stick (tough to find suitable veins to administer chemo), and the frequency and duration of chemotherapy cycles needed.

- **Orally**: As a student, I never thought that chemotherapy could be given as a pill. That all changed in 2001, when the FDA approved a drug called capecitabine (Xeloda) as the first oral chemotherapy drug for colorectal cancer. Chemotherapy as a pill? That was revolutionary at the time. Now, most new cancer drugs that get approved are pills. This is understandable as many patients prefer oral drugs because they are easy to administer and many can be taken at home, minimizing visits to the oncologist's office. However, side effects can be as bad with oral pills as they are with IV chemotherapy. Not all chemotherapy drugs are available by mouth, and similarly, not all chemotherapy drugs are available intravenously.

- **Under the skin**: Some chemotherapy drugs can be given as an injection under the skin. The needle used is often very small, similar to those used to administer insulin to diabetic patients.

- **Through the muscle**: Several chemotherapy drugs are given this way; often, they cause some muscle soreness and maybe a bit of redness and inflammation on the skin where the injection was given.

- **Through the spinal canal**: Chemotherapy administered through the spinal canal is called intrathecal therapy. The thought of injecting chemotherapy through the spinal canal can make anyone cringe, but sometimes, this is necessary depending on the type of cancer. This can be done at the bedside or in the office, but sometimes, a radiologist is needed to direct where exactly to inject the chemotherapy. The patient lies on their side or sits upright and bends slightly so that the space between the vertebrae opens up enough to make the injection easier. What is important here is for the patient to lie flat for a while after the procedure is over, typically for about 30 minutes but sometimes an hour. This usually reduces the chance of developing a headache that can result from the spinal tap.

- **A pump**: Sometimes chemotherapy needs to be given continuously. The chemotherapy drug is placed inside a pump that delivers the drug in prespecified intervals based on how the pump is programmed. Before these pumps became available, patients were admitted to the hospital to undergo the infusion, but patients can now receive infusional chemotherapy in the comfort of their home. Sometimes, these pumps can be internal and placed under the skin surgically, and the chemotherapy is delivered through a catheter to the area needed. Most often, this is used in certain circumstances when colon cancer has gone to the liver, and we need to give regional chemotherapy to the liver area where the cancer had spread. Alternatively, the pump can be external and placed in a fanny pack or a shoulder pack. In general, these would be battery operated and require a visiting nurse to initiate or disconnect.

Dose and Trade-Offs

"How much chemotherapy will I receive and for how long?" he asked.

"Well, it depends," I answered as I sensed his confusion. "For your chemo regimen, most drugs are given based on height and weight."

Basically, the doses of many intravenous chemotherapy drugs are calculated based on a formula called body surface area (BSA). Some drugs are given based entirely on weight (mg/kg). Others can be given as a fixed dose, although the latter is common when giving oral chemotherapy or small molecules (please see chapter 13 on targeted therapy). As we described when discussing clinical trials, phase 1 studies are designed to find out the proper dose for future studies and subsequently for routine clinical care.

Some might suggest that dosing chemotherapy this way is totally acceptable. Others disagree and propose that we need to better understand how drugs are metabolized within one's body and that we need to investigate the likelihood that a patient might respond to a drug before administering it. This led to the birth of the field of pharmacogenomics, which uses information about the patient's genetic makeup to select the drugs and doses that are likely to work best in this particular individual for this particular disease. Sounds too good to be true. Maybe, but as this field continues to evolve, we still use the older methods to find out the proper dosing and schedules of chemotherapies.

Commonly, in older patients or in those who might have suboptimal liver or kidney function, the doses of whichever chemotherapy drugs being prescribed might need to be adjusted to minimize side effects and maximize potential benefit.

When giving chemotherapy intravenously, doctors can ensure that the patient is indeed getting their treatment as they are right there in the office receiving it. When prescribing oral chemotherapy, doctors fear that their patients might forget to take their pills on time, and adherence might become an issue. Figuring out how to overcome barriers to nonadherence is a topic that is front and center of "healthcare delivery" science.

There are economic issues as well when deciding how to give chemotherapy. Patients have certain co-pays and financial responsibilities, which differ based on whether the drug is given orally or by vein. Also, there are differences based on whether the drugs are given in the office or at the hospital. These details are beyond the scope of this book but are critical to discuss with the treating physician and the financial counselor at the treating facility. My advice for patients is to always ask questions and get as many details as possible.

Take-Home Points

- Chemotherapy given after a definitive treatment of the cancer is called adjuvant therapy.

- Chemotherapy given before the definitive treatment of the cancer is called neoadjuvant chemotherapy.

- Sometimes, chemotherapy is given as the sole modality to cure the cancer (such as in some forms of lymphomas), but other times it is given as part of a larger protocol that includes surgery, radiation, and other modalities.

- Commonly, chemotherapy is given just to alleviate symptoms and/or to increase survival, but not to cure the disease. In these situations, we label it as palliative chemotherapy.

- There are many types of chemotherapeutic agents that work through different mechanisms of action. Please ask your doctor what you're taking and, if you're curious, how they work.

- Chemotherapy can be given in different ways: intravenously, orally, under the skin, through the muscle, through the spinal canal, or via a pump.

- Oral chemotherapy can have many side effects. The route by which you receive the chemotherapy does not always dictate the type or severity of side effects.

CHAPTER 11

Treating the Cancer: Radiation Therapy

The more violent the storm,
the quicker it passes.

—*Paulo Coelho*

THE FIRST THING I thought about when I started learning about radiation therapy was fumes and nuclear explosions. Growing up, I couldn't wrap my head around what radiation therapy was. I was in Syria in medical school when the nuclear accident at Chernobyl happened in 1986. In my simple mind, radiation was synonymous with something ominous and dangerous, just like Chernobyl. Now, I am confident that many patients feel the same and conjure images of burning ovens, nuclear reactors, and other gloomy ideas when pondering about radiation treatments. It's why I wanted to learn about the field—so that I could explain it to my patients in simplified terms.

It turns out that radiation as a modality existed for hundreds of years, and some trace it back to earlier than the 1900s. In fact, X-rays were discovered in 1895 by Wilhelm Roentgen, who won the first

Nobel Prize in Physics. Roentgen's discovery was incidental, but the field of radiation therapy never looked back and continued to progress exponentially, especially after Marie Curie coined the term "radioactivity" in 1898. Marie Curie was the first woman to ever win a Nobel Prize and the first and only woman to win the Nobel Prize twice. Although she was born in Poland, she did most of her work in France, where she was naturalized as a French citizen and was a professor at the University of Paris. She is famous for developing mobile radiography units that she drove to provide X-ray services to field hospitals during World War I.

My patient was very scared, and I could tell that there was a lot that he didn't know. While there is so much information on the internet, nothing replaces putting the trust in a physician who can separate the signal from the noise, who can help explain a complex field and what it means for each patient. So, when I saw the look of fear in my patient's eyes, I knew he was terrified. He was diagnosed with rectal cancer at the age of 52. He was initially referred to a surgeon who told him that he needed to see me first, as he would benefit from receiving chemotherapy and radiation therapy before undergoing the surgery.

I explained to him that chemotherapy and radiation can prevent the cancer from recurring and make the tumor smaller and the surgery even better. The chemotherapy would make the radiation more effective in shrinking the cancer.

I told him, "We know also that if you have these before surgery, you would fare better than surgery alone. Patients who get chemo and radiation before surgery for your type of cancer live longer than patients who have surgery alone."

He asked, "How long would I have that for?"

"About six weeks or so. You will need radiation therapy every day from Monday through Friday as you also get the chemotherapy. I will supervise your treatment and the chemo you will receive, but you'll need to see another doctor who will be responsible for delivering the radiation therapy to you. That doctor is a radiation oncologist, and that is their specialty."

He was not thrilled at the suggestion he would need yet another doctor. This reaction is not uncommon. Overnight, a patient goes from having one or no doctor to a team of doctors with varied expertise and specialties. Being overwhelmed is the norm, and our role is to ensure that this feeling is minimized, which best achieved by spending more time with the patient and simplifying the process. I did my best to explain everything to him.

"The radiation oncologist will determine how much radiation you will receive and where to aim it," I said. "Think of the radiation beams as rays that target the tumor and kill the cancer cells where they are. They are precise, so the team will decide the actual area that needs targeting, and they will do their best to protect the normal and healthy tissues around it so that you experience as few side effects as possible."

He protested, "All I hear is horror stories about radiation therapy."

He is not alone in having heard scary things about radiation. When talking radiation therapy, I often tell patients to think about how the skin gets damaged when exposed to the sun for a long time. I then suggest that radiation therapy is delivering high-energy X-ray (similar to the rays of the sun) to areas where the cancer is located with the aim of destroying these cancer cells. This is very different from chemotherapy, where the drugs are given to affect cancer cells wherever they are. Radiation therapy is designed generally to affect one location. It might impact surrounding normal and healthy tissue, however; therefore, extreme precautions are taken to minimize the extent of possible collateral damage. Radiation, similar to chemotherapy, does affect the DNA of cancer cells, so they stop growing and multiplying. Radiation is delivered in a daily dose known as a *fraction*.

As you could imagine, radiation therapy can be given in various ways, but it's fair to divide delivery based on whether it is from the outside in (external) or the inside out (internal).

External Radiation Therapy

The machine used for external radiation therapy is called a *linear accelerator* (or LINAC). The machine delivers beams of X-ray. The dose is calculated by the radiation oncologist and the medical physicist, who is more familiar with the machine software, which is extremely precise and is adjusted to deliver the desired dose to the specified location. The first step in any radiation therapy is to meet with the radiation oncologist. Then, a planning session/visit, also known as a *simulation session*, is performed. This session is usually performed on a specialized CT scanner and sometimes on MRI. The idea here is to use CT scan or MRI-based images to create a three-dimensional model of the patient, their tumor, and the surrounding organs. During the planning visit, the technician places skin markings (we call them *tattoos*) that help align the radiation in future sessions to the exact desired location. The subsequent visit is when the first radiation session takes place. Sometimes, patients may wait one to two weeks after the planning appointment to start therapy, as it does take time to map out and plan the radiation fields to make sure they meet safety criteria and to perform the necessary double checks on the plan. This helps to deliver the radiation more precisely, and hopefully reduces side effects to the surrounding healthy areas.

There are different types of external radiation that are worth mentioning, but the general principle is to always maximize radiation delivery to the target while minimizing any radiation to the surrounding healthy tissue. In all types of radiation, multiple radiation beams are directed at the tumor, and where the beams all meet is where the maximum amount of radiation is given.

- **Three-dimensional conformal radiation therapy (3D-CRT):** The idea here is to use radiation beams that are shaped to the tumor while protecting nearby organs. This is an advancement over two-dimensional radiation. The planning session CT scan or MRI-based images are used to create a three-dimensional picture of the tumor and surrounding organs. This helps in targeting the radiation delivery and reducing side effects to the surrounding healthy areas.

- **Intensity-modulated radiation therapy (IMRT):** Think of this as an enhancement to 3D-CRT because it offers more control over every single beam that is being delivered. It allows us to provide higher doses of radiation to the tumor while adjusting the beams to reduce the strength of the radiation within each beam, thus protecting normal tissues. It is precise and preferred over other methods, and it requires an entire team to ensure adequate delivery.

- **Tomotherapy/volumetric modulated arc therapy (VMAT):** This is a form of IMRT that is delivered by rotating the machine around the patient. It also allows the medical team to adjust the dose and direction of the radiation beams to match the size and shape of the tumor being targeted. Its advantages include better shaping of the radiation for irregularly shaped tumors. Similar to standard IMRT, it may reduce radiation to normal tissues, which could translate into fewer side effects.

- **Electron radiation:** Electrons are another form of radiation that are given to superficial tumors, such as skin cancers or scars after breast cancer surgery, often in benign conditions such as keloids.

- **Proton beam therapy**: X-rays are not used in proton beam therapy but rather charged particles that we call *protons*, which can kill the cancer cells. Proponents of proton therapy argue that it delivers more radiation to the cancer and little, if any, outside of the cancer. Opponents argue that we don't know if it is better than the other techniques I have described, and it is more expensive. Sometimes, protons will allow less radiation to be delivered to the healthy tissue, but it depends on the location being treated. Nowadays, more centers in the United States have these proton therapy capabilities to be able to offer this technology to patients, particularly children with cancer. I have seen my colleagues in the radiation oncology recommend it in some pediatric cancers or in cancers that are close to sensitive areas in the body, like the spinal cord or the eyes. The machine used is called a *cyclotron* or *synchrotron*; it speeds up the protons, creating more energy to help the protons travel to the desired depth inside the body where they can reach the tumor and deliver the desired radiation dose. The radiation beam can penetrate to a certain depth in the patient and stops giving radiation at a certain point, so this reduces scatter radiation within the patient. Usual side effects are fatigue and skin changes comparable to all the other types of radiation—nothing surprising.

  I am not a radiation oncologist, but I know many who are, and I believe that this proton therapy approach is divisive. Many radiation oncologists are proponents, and equally, many are against. Not every center or hospital in the United States has proton therapy capabilities, but if I were a betting man, more will have this technology in the near future. For now, doctors must decide the most appropriate type of radiation for each patient.

Because of their targeted nature, IMRT, VMAT, and proton beam therapy are commonly used on areas that previously would have been irradiated.

With most modern radiation therapy, special images or scans are taken before each treatment to make sure the alignment to the tumor is appropriate. This is known as *image-guided radiation therapy* (IGRT), and it is performed for all the external beam radiation modalities mentioned here.

- **Radiosurgery**: While we call this radio "surgery," it requires no hospital stay or anesthesia. This is done as a one-time, single large dose of radiation therapy, although sometimes it can be given over few doses and days. Theoretically, it can cure tumors that would have otherwise required surgery in situations where the doctors feel that surgery is too risky or not possible, and that doing radiation is safer. When given to areas in the brain, we call this *stereotactic radiosurgery*, or SRS, and when given to other areas in the body, we label this as *stereotactic body radiotherapy*, or SBRT. There are certain requirements to optimize SRS or SBRT, such as the size, location, and number of tumors. Generally, this kind of radiation is given for several days with larger doses each day. What we are doing here is literally ablating the tumor with higher doses of radiation delivered precisely to where the tumor is located.
  - *Gamma Knife*: Probably the easiest and fastest way to explain Gamma Knife is to think of it as a CyberKnife (described below) but delivered to tumors and abnormalities within the brain. Usually, about 200 tiny beams of radiation are delivered to the tumor or other targets with submillimeter accuracy. These beams all meet in one place to collectively deliver a large, effective dose of radiation. This treatment is delivered generally in one outpatient session but can also be

given in multiple sessions. Healthy tissues for the most part are spared any radiation or get only minimal radiation. Basically, the Gamma Knife allows an alternative in any scenario where the doctor, the patient, or both wish to avoid an operation to the brain. Because the treatment is given to the brain tissue, some swelling might develop but could take months; this can be treated with anti-inflammatory medicines. Also, fatigue and nausea might develop, and certainly skin and hair changes can occur since the treatment is delivered through the skull.

o *CyberKnife*: CyberKnife is a brand name type of SRS/SBRT. This idea is credited to Dr. John Adler, a professor and neurosurgeon at Stanford University. He did a fellowship in Sweden under the direction of Dr. Lars Leksell, who founded the concept of radiosurgery and the Gamma Knife machine for treating brain tumors. Adler developed a noninvasive robotic system that improves treatment accuracy by using image-guided technology and computer-controlled robotics to continually track and correct delivery of radiation based on the size of the tumor and the patient's movements. This precision allows the doctors to use CyberKnife anywhere in the body. I don't think patients need to spend a lot of time understanding the mechanics of these machines; even non-radiation oncologists don't understand all the mechanics. What must be understood is that there are options to eradicate tumors using radiation. Surgery has not been compared with SRS in all tumors, because as you could imagine, it would be impossible to compare. Often, if a patient can undergo surgery, that is what they choose, while SRS is reserved for patients who cannot undergo surgery. So, SRS is delivering higher doses of radiation during a short period of time, while traditional radiation is delivering lower doses over a longer time.

Internal Radiation Therapy

Internal radiation therapy is what we call *brachytherapy*. It is giving radiation from the inside of the organ targeted out. So, naturally, it requires placing radioactive material inside the organ where cancer cells are growing. These implants can be temporary or permanent, and placing them often requires being in the hospital for a day or so. The temporary implants are delivered through special catheters that give radiation either over a few minutes or a few days. The permanent implants are steel seeds that carry radioactive material, and they deliver radiation around the implanted area. Because the seeds can exert radiation outside the body, very specific safety measures are implemented so that people living with the patient are not harmed. These seeds lose their radioactivity with time, but they stay where they were implanted and can be viewed on X-rays.

Other Forms of Radiation Therapy

- **Radioimmunotherapy**: This type of radiation uses an antibody, which is a protein that attaches to a target on the surface of the cancer cell, to deliver the radiation directly to the tumor.

- **Intraoperative radiation**: We are sometimes able to give radiation to the tumor during the surgery. The surgeon moves the healthy organs out of the way so that planned radiation (external or internal) can be given.

- **Total body irradiation (TBI)**: This is usually done as part of the preparation to undergo some forms of bone marrow transplantation (or what we now call *stem cell transplantation*). It delivers radiation to the entire body, as the name implies.

Goals of Radiation Therapy

There are two main goals when we decide on treating cancer. We aim either to eradicate and cure it if we can, or to control it when cure is not possible. Radiation can serve one of these two purposes depending on the disease, the stage, and the goals of care dictated by each patient and their medical team.

Curing the Cancer

- Some cancers can be cured by radiation therapy alone. Even in my own field of lymphoma, radiation used to be given as the sole modality to cure certain types of lymphomas. Some tumors are sensitive to radiation and when in early stage can be cured by radiation alone. Examples are small early cancers in the head and neck areas (lip, tongue, etc.) or early-stage follicular lymphoma, among others.

- Sometimes, radiation therapy is given as part of a program that includes chemotherapy.
  - Radiation can be given in conjunction with chemotherapy. So, the patient is getting the chemotherapy intravenously or by mouth at the same time they are getting radiation. Usually, the chemotherapy here is labeled as *radiosensitizer*, meaning that at the doses administered, the chemotherapy will make the cancer tissue more susceptible to the effects of radiation.
  - Radiation can be given at the end of the chemotherapy (we call this *consolidation* or *adjuvant radiotherapy*). Some women with breast cancer, for example, receive radiation after they finish chemotherapy and surgery for their early stage disease. Radiation here is part of the adjuvant program.
  - Sometimes, we give radiation before surgery to shrink the tumor (*neoadjuvant radiation*), although often we add chemother-

apy to radiation in this setting. Patients with rectal cancer routinely undergo radiation before surgery.

Controlling the Cancer

- When we cannot cure the cancer, we can give radiation therapy to mitigate the pain or other symptoms, such as bleeding in certain areas. Cancers that spread to the bones can cause a lot of pain, and giving radiation to these bony areas can relieve the pain significantly. This is what we call *palliative radiation*, as we are palliating the cancer symptoms. We recognize that we cannot cure the cancer, but we can still shrink the tumor to make the patient feel better. Other situations where radiation can help include relieving pressure from tumors that create spinal cord compression or other neurological symptoms. Occasionally, we give chemotherapy in conjunction with radiation, even when the goal is palliative.

- Even when we cannot cure the cancer, giving the radiation alongside chemotherapy in certain conditions can prolong life and help control the disease. For example, many brain tumors are not curable, but giving the radiation with chemotherapy in that setting controls the tumor and prolongs survival.

Side Effects of Radiation Therapy

- **Short-term effects**: These are the side effects you might experience as you're going through radiation therapy or shortly thereafter. One thing about radiation is that it continues to exert its activity even after the treatment has been completed since the cancer cells are continuing to die off.
  - *Skin changes*: These can include redness, itching, and sometimes blisters. Doctors prescribe creams or ointments that

can alleviate these symptoms. Often, these improve gradually after completion of therapy, but sometimes the color changes and dryness persists.

o *Fatigue*: Fatigue is one of the most common effects of radiation. Although the fatigue is mild to moderate, I always advise my patients to try exercising, even if it's just long or short walks. In my opinion, being active is the best remedy to combat fatigue, which is expected the longer the radiation course continues.

o *Mouth sores and dry mouth*: These occur anytime radiation is given to areas where the mouth and throat are in the field. Think of some of the head and neck cancers as an example. Tooth decay could occur, and many doctors ask for a dental consult before treatment so that decays are treated ahead of radiation.

o *Swallowing difficulty*: If radiation is given to the chest area where the esophagus is going through, sores within the esophagus can develop, which can lead to difficulty swallowing, and, of course, weight loss. Doctors try to combat this by asking patients to use nutritional supplements that are easy to swallow, although there are times when temporary feeding tubes are required.

o *GI side effects*: These depend on where the radiation is being delivered. Esophageal pain or trouble swallowing might occur when radiation is given to the head and neck area or to the chest. Nausea and vomiting can occur, and some patients lose weight. Radiation to the bowels can lead to diarrhea and pain and redness in the rectal region that requires topical treatment.

o *Hair loss*: This depends on whether the radiation is given to areas where there is hair growth. Radiation to the chest, for example, might cause hair loss on the chest or back but would not impact hair on the head.

○ *Bladder irritation*: This can cause urinary complaints and, as you might have guessed, occurs when the radiation is given to the pelvis and the bladder is not spared completely, which is not unusual.

○ *Lowered blood counts*: These occur more often when chemotherapy is administered alongside radiation. Lower white counts can lead to infections, and patients might need transfusions if their red cells and/or platelets are too low.

- **Long-term and/or midterm effects**
  ○ The side effect that we fear the most is future cancer that develops years after the radiation is complete. There are many cancers that can develop because of radiation or chemotherapy, and it is important that patients are monitored for years so that doctors are aware of any changes that might suggest new cancers. Some of the cancers can be bone marrow cancers if we are giving radiation to the hip bones and pelvis. By getting one cancer, patients are also predisposed to other cancers, so continued checkups with your doctors are important.

  ○ Radiation to the chest can cause pulmonary fibrosis (lung scarring). Basically, the lungs become stiff, and patients can get short of breath and have a cough and other respiratory symptoms. Not uncommonly, patients can develop a condition called *radiation pneumonitis*—basically, this is an inflammation in the lungs from radiation that is treated with steroids.

  ○ Heart issues and coronary artery disease can occur when radiation is given to the left side of the chest. These can be magnified if radiation is given alongside a chemotherapy drug that can also affect the heart.

○ I have seen "radiation necrosis": this is dead tissue from radiation, but because of its location it can cause significant side effects. The brain area is usually the most vulnerable to this toxicity, but the good news is that there are treatments for this problem. Radiation necrosis usually is not seen in most other parts of the body.

My patient asked me, "Could you please list all side effects that I might encounter?"

"How about this?" I replied. "I will tell you the most common ones, but let's not do a list. If I give you a list and you experience something that is not on the list, you're going to assume that it's not related. I'd rather you call me and let me know how you feel and share any of your symptoms, and let me decide if it is related to the treatment or not."

"I don't want to bother you," he responded.

"It is better for us to know," I reassured him. "Call me or my nurse, but keep us informed. It is impossible to list every possible problem that might develop."

This was always the principle I used when I was seeing patients. How can we practically list every single possible side effect? What if a patient develops something that is not listed? Practically, I always advised and described the common side effects, alerting patients to keep the line of communication open. So, the list I just provided is a sample of the most common ones, and some might have been missed. Doctors must stay informed and aware of any of the side effects patients experience. Not all patients are the same, and similar therapy can have different effects on different patients.

Take-Home Points

- Radiation therapy is a modality to control the cancer by delivering beams on the cancer growth, killing the cells by damaging the DNA and thereby preventing the cells from replicating.

- There are different ways of delivering radiation therapy; your radiation oncologist is the doctor who determines the best way of giving radiation, the dose, and the location.

- Sometimes radiation alone can cure the cancer, but often it is given with chemotherapy, as together these can have a better effect on the cancer. Your radiation oncologist and medical oncologist will confer to decide.

- On occasion, radiation is given to control the symptoms that cancer is causing, especially alleviating cancer pain. Radiation in these situations won't cure the cancer but likely will make you feel better.

- Your team will make every effort to minimize the normal tissue and normal cells from being exposed to radiation so as to minimize side effects.

- There are short-term and long-term side effects of radiation; please make sure you discuss these with your doctors.

CHAPTER 12

Treating the Cancer: Hormonal Therapy

Sometimes life hits you in the head with a brick.
Don't lose faith.

—*Steve Jobs*

WALKING THE HALLWAYS of the University of Chicago, you're often faced with portraits of luminaries who have left their fingerprints on all disciplines in life. One of these is the picture of Charles Huggins (or as his colleagues called him, Chuck). I had learned and read about Huggins's research and accomplishments as arguably the scientist who changed how we treat prostate cancer by depriving the body from testosterone, the male hormone. Huggins showed that some cancer cells depend on these hormones to survive, grow, and multiply. Moreover, along with his collaborators, he showed that depriving cancer cells of these hormonal signals can help slow the spread of metastases. His work won him the Cameron Prize for Therapeutics at the University of Edinburgh and the Nobel Prize in Physiology or Medicine in 1966.

Huggins worked with a medical student, Clarence Hodges, on investigating how best to control prostatic tumors. Early in 1941, the duet studied eight patients with prostate cancer that had gone to the bones, investigating the effect of pharmaceutical or medical castration using estrogens or removing the testes, and how that could lower blood markers that were hypothesized to be produced from the prostate. The markers indeed decreased, followed by clinical improvement. This discovery was among the first to recognize that hormones play a role in the development of some cancers.

Huggins's expertise in prostate cancer and how it can be dependent on testosterone led him in the 1950s to study breast cancer. He showed that some breast cancers are dependent on estrogens and can improve by removing the hormonal source (ovaries and the adrenal glands). Arguably, these were the initial discoveries that led to dividing breast cancers into estrogen receptor–positive and estrogen receptor–negative diseases.

Hormones are substances that the human body produces from various organs, and they control specific functions by affecting how certain types of cells work and behave. Most people are familiar with the thyroid hormone, maybe because thyroid disorders are common. If there is too much of the thyroid hormone, the patient can lose weight, develop palpitations, encounter diarrhea, and have a whole lot of symptoms that are reversed by decreasing the levels of that hormone. Different symptoms develop when there is too little of the thyroid hormone in the body.

It turns out that some cancers are dependent on hormones, meaning they grow and multiply because of the presence of these hormones. Cancers that are dependent on hormones can improve by blocking the production of such hormones. Hormonal therapies are drugs that either stop the body entirely from secreting these hormones, block their production partially, prevent the hormones from attaching to the cancer cells to make them grow, or alter the produced hormone so that it doesn't perform the function it was destined to.

How and When Is Hormonal Therapy Given?

Generally, any treatment that we give before the "definitive local treatment" of the cancer is called neoadjuvant therapy. Any treatment given after is labeled adjuvant therapy. Definitive treatment is often surgery, although sometimes it can be radiation therapy. Overall, adjuvant and neoadjuvant treatments are given when the goal of therapy is cure. Hormonal therapies have been given in both states—neoadjuvant and adjuvant. However, there are many situations when cure is not possible, and hormonal therapy is given as a method to control the cancer; when so, it can be the sole treatment or administered as part of a larger program.

Conversations with patients and families about hormonal treatments are never easy, especially in younger individuals. I recall meeting a 55-year-old man who had prostate cancer that had spread to the bones. It was clear that he needed hormonal therapy that would deprive his body of testosterone.

> *CN:* Your prostate cancer is driven by testosterone that is mainly produced by the testes. We need to block that. Think of the prostate cancer as a car that needs fuel to keep running and spreading from one organ to another. What I am recommending is to stop the fuel supply. This way, the car stops running, at least for a while.
>
> *Patient:* OK, so the cancer stops growing and spreading?
>
> *CN:* Not forever, but hopefully for a long time.
>
> *Patient:* How do we do that?
>
> *CN:* There are two ways. We can perform surgery and remove the testicles. This takes out the main production source of testosterone. It is an easy surgery that is performed by a urologist. The

other way if you choose no surgery is to give you shots in the muscle or under the skin that block your body's ability to produce testosterone. These shots can be given monthly, every three months, or even every six months depending on which kind we use.

While decades ago, removing the testicles surgically was commonly used to deprive the body of testosterone in metastatic prostate cancer, it is rarely done now and has been largely replaced by these shots. The surgery, called orchiectomy, is an outpatient procedure and is considered simple and inexpensive. Its major drawback is that it is permanent as we can't reverse course once surgery is performed. When shots are given for that same purpose, stopping them might reverse course and testosterone production can return, albeit that return might take longer in some patients than others. In a 2020 report, 33,585 patients with metastatic prostate cancer were investigated. There was a significant decline in surgical castration from 8.6% in 2004 to 3.1% in 2014. It is not clear why fewer orchiectomies occur, but likely there is an economic component as manufacturers of these drugs (the shots) sustain a steady stream of revenue since these injections are continued permanently. Moreover, patients likely prefer a reversible approach; they can reverse the castration by stopping the shots should their goals of care change. The shots essentially cause a type of "menopause" for men who may experience hot flashes, fatigue, and possibly bone density loss. Some patients gain weight, and occasionally the breasts might slightly enlarge and become painful.

The most important part of giving hormonal therapy is to be vigilant to potential adverse events. While some suggest that hormonal therapy is easier and better tolerated than chemotherapy, for example, I would offer that the type of side effects patients encounter is different, and being familiar with these should put patients at an advantage. Other side effects of these hormonal injections for prostate cancer are a lack of sexual desire, erectile dysfunction, depression, and loss of muscle mass. The most important side effects to watch for are cardiac as there have been some reports that these injections can increase risk of cardiac disease. This is essential as prostate cancer is diagnosed and treated in older men, where risk factors for cardiac disease might be more prevalent. There are many published reports on risks associated with androgen deprivation therapy (ADT) and cardiac diseases (see the sources at the end of the book for more comprehensive studies), but assessing the risk estimate has not been consistent across all analyses. Most studies do not suggest increased risk in mortality but more risk with arrythmias, heart failure, and sclerosis of the arteries. The hypothesis is that these risks stem from weight gain, elevated lipids, lack of activity, and other risk factors. I keep this issue front and center and work with my patients on reducing cardiac risk factors, staying vigilant to any possible cardiac problem that might emerge.

Hormonal therapies are often used in treating the following cancers:

Prostate cancer: When hormonal therapy is needed for the reasons I described, we call this "androgen suppression or deprivation therapy." If orchiectomy is not chosen, then we can prescribe injectable drugs called luteinizing hormone–releasing hormone (LHRH) agonists to lower testosterone. Examples of these include leuprolide (Lupron), goserelin (Zoladex), and triptorelin (Trelstar). When initially given, these drugs can cause a slight surge in testosterone, commonly referred to as a "tumor flare," but we can suppress the flare by giving oral medications alongside the injections, called antiandrogens.

There are also the LHRH antagonists; these work a bit differently but also lower testosterone levels. Examples include degarelix (Firmagon) and relugolix (Orgovyx).

As I was telling my patient all these side effects he could encounter, he interrupted, "Could you please just tell me what I can do about it?"

"You must try to exercise despite the fatigue; this will help your muscle mass and elevate your mood," I responded. "There are medications to treat the hot flashes, and if there is breast tenderness, we can try to give some radiation therapy to that area, which will minimize the pain. We will do bone density testing and certainly make sure you have the best bone health by taking the needed supplements, such as calcium and others."

The way these LHRH agonists and antagonists work is by stopping the production of testosterone from the testicles, but guess what? Sometimes testosterone and the male hormones can be produced from other sources, usually the adrenal glands. Because of that, drugs were developed to prevent these sources outside the testicles from producing the androgens and testosterone. An example is abiraterone (Zytiga), which blocks an enzyme (called CYP17) that helps the cells make androgens. Another older drug that could do that is ketoconazole, which is normally an antifungal therapy but also blocks the adrenal glands from producing androgens.

Antiandrogens are drugs that don't prevent the production of androgens but rather prevent them from working after they are already produced. It turns out that androgens need to attach to a protein on the surface of the prostate cancer cell for them to work. So, if we can prevent the androgens from attaching to their receptor, we can hopefully slow prostate cancer growth. In medical textbooks, these are called androgen receptor antagonists and include bicalutamide, flutamide, or nilutamide, all taken by mouth.

Recall the tumor flare we described earlier; the doctor sometimes starts these antiandrogens a couple of weeks before the LHRH shots to prevent the flare. After that, the doctor might either recommend continuing both or stopping the oral pill.

There are new versions of these antiandrogens. Examples are enzalutamide (Xtandi), apalutamide (Erleada), and darolutamide (Nubeqa). These are all taken by mouth, and they are theorized to be better than the older versions in certain circumstances.

What is important is that these drugs do not affect testosterone production from the testicles, so patients must continue LHRH shots even if they are getting treatment with antiandrogens or with the drugs that prevent their production from the adrenal glands. The adrenal gland can produce other hormones, so when we use drugs that suppress its function, we must replace the substances that we still want produced. For example, men who are on abiraterone must take prednisone.

One of my patients who was very knowledgeable about medicine was diagnosed with prostate cancer a few years before I started seeing him and was getting one of these injections I mentioned earlier. He came to see me because the urologist who was treating him told him that these shots were no longer working. I recall seeing him the first time around and how disappointed he was that the shots stopped working. But the cancer cells can start to outsmart the medications by growing in a way that no longer requires testosterone. And then it is time to find another treatment path.

I told my patient, "When prostate cancer needs testosterone to grow, we call the disease hormone sensitive. Eventually, it becomes hormone insensitive or castration resistant. I think this is where you are now, and we need to discuss various options and next steps."

Prostate cancer is hormonally driven, and that knowledge was a fascinating discovery at the time. But, like all cancers that are driven by hormones, eventually it stops responding to hormonal therapy. In the castration-sensitive stage of this disease, physicians contemplate how much suppression of testosterone is needed. Some use the injections alone while others use the injections plus antiandrogens. In medical books, this debate is called androgen deprivation therapy (ADT) versus complete androgen blockade (CAB). I don't have a real preference for one over the other, and the exact pros and cons of one approach versus another is beyond the scope of this book, but it is an important topic to bring up with your doctor if applicable. Another debate centers on whether patients should undergo continuous ADT (basically, getting the injections forever until they stop working) or intermittent

ADT (getting the shots until testosterone levels in the blood go very low, at which point we stop the shots and resume them when the levels go up). Of course, the rationale for the intermittent approach is that the breaks allow for fewer side effects and maybe the return of some sexual function temporarily, which might improve quality of life.

In recent developments for hormone-sensitive prostate cancer, patients are offered ADT plus additional therapies as an upfront approach, which has been shown to improve survival. Some patients receive ADT plus chemotherapy, while others receive ADT plus one of the novel hormonal treatments (abiraterone or enzalutamide). While treating patients with more upfront approaches may make them live longer, such approaches might not be for everyone as there are trade-offs of possible side effects. Discussing pros and cons and individualizing this is essential.

Breast cancer: My mom was once on hormonal replacement therapy (HRT). There is a chance that some women readers of this book were once on HRT as well. Why? Because at some point there was a suggestion that we could combat menopausal symptoms by giving women estrogens or estrogens plus progestins. In the 1990s, a study called the Women's Health Initiative was started, and as part of this study investigators attempted to answer the question of whether HRT could ease menopausal symptoms and improve bone health. I vividly recall that my own mother had terrible menopausal symptoms and her bones became fragile, so anything that could possibly help was welcome, although she was placed on HRT by her doctors without participating in any study or trial. In 1996, a similar study, asking a similar question, was started in the United Kingdom called the Million Women Study.

The Women's Health Initiative study was halted in 2002 when it was discovered that women who were on HRT had increased risk of breast cancer and heart disease. The link between estrogen and breast cancer was further solidified, and many women, including my mother, came off HRT after these results were publicized. We had known previously that some breast cancers can be treated with hormonal manipulation by giving affected individuals therapies that block hormones from attaching to their receptors on the surface of breast cancer cells. Of course, not all women will have these receptors. These hormonal therapies have traditionally worked only in individuals whose breast cancer cells were estrogen positive. It is estimated that two-thirds of breast cancers are receptor positive.

What types of hormonal therapies are given in breast cancer? Common sense dictates that we give drugs that either block the receptors or prevent estrogen production from its sources.

There are several drugs that can block the estrogen receptors. I came to learn about these drugs, what they did, and how they did it during my fellowship at Northwestern University. I was doing basic science research in the laboratory of Dr. Steven Rosen, whom I consider a true mentor and a friend, and would come across others who were doing research in the laboratory of Dr. V. Craig Jordan, the "Father of Tamoxifen."

Tamoxifen was first synthesized in 1962 by scientists at a British company called Imperial Chemical Industries, now called AstraZeneca. The drug was originally found to have contraceptive effects in rats; it is why tamoxifen was initially being developed as a morning-after pill. In the 1970s, however, it was found to have the opposite effects in humans; indeed, it increased fertility and ovulation in women. It was subsequently studied for breast cancer because of its antiestrogen effects on cells that had the estrogen receptor. Interestingly, tamoxifen was found to stimulate the estrogen activity in the uterus, and it's why it was renamed selective estrogen receptor modulator, or SERM. Dr. Jordan's work was mainly on SERMs. Tamoxifen was approved in 1978 for treating breast cancer receptor-positive disease that had spread elsewhere, but subsequently, it was also used for preventing breast cancer in women at high risk for developing the disease. Subsequent studies showed that tamoxifen can reduce the risk of breast cancer recurrence in patients diagnosed with receptor-positive disease and the risk of developing breast cancer in the healthy breast. Because of how tamoxifen works, it is usually given only to women who are premenopausal. Also, because of how it works on the uterus, women must be monitored for the possibility of developing uterine cancer if they have been on tamoxifen for a long time. I always quizzed my students on the top three side effects of tamoxifen: uterine cancer, blood clots, and vision problems, mainly early cataracts. Of course, there are other side effects to watch for, such as hot flashes since the drug prevents the work of estrogen.

Tamoxifen is credited with saving millions of lives. Due to his discoveries and dedication to the field, Dr. Jordan was elected to the National Academy of Sciences in 2009 and won the American Cancer Society Medal of Honor in 2002, among other awards too numerous to count. In 2002, he received the Order of the British Empire from Queen Elizabeth II for services to international breast cancer research. The queen appointed him Companion of the Most Distinguished Order of St. Michael and St. George. Tamoxifen remains one of the world's most successful drugs against cancer and is on the World Health Organization's list of essential medicines.

There are other hormonal drugs that break down the estrogen receptor. The most well-known one is called fulvestrant (Faslodex). It is a selective estrogen receptor degrader (SERD), but because of how it works, it can be given to women in menopause or in premenopause as long as the premenopausal women receive drugs that induce them into menopause.

Now, there are other hormonal drugs that treat breast cancer but through reducing the levels of estrogens in the blood. The most notable ones are these called aromatase inhibitors, or AIs.

AIs stop the production of estrogens in the body from sources outside the ovaries. Estrogens are usually produced in the ovaries, but in menopause, when ovaries are no longer functioning, estrogens are made in the body fat through an enzyme called aromatase. These drugs inhibit the work of that enzyme, leading to lower production of estrogens. They are used in women who develop breast cancer in the postmenopausal phase, but they can be used in the premenopausal condition if women are induced into menopause. There are several known drugs that belong to this class: anastrozole (Arimidex), letrozole (Femara), and exemestane (Aromasin). Because of how AIs work, doctors are always concerned about how these medications might affect bone health and make the bones thinner, so doctors often prescribe treatment to strengthen the bones and periodically check bone health using a bone density test. The other side effects that patients need to be aware of are muscle and joint aches and pains; these are almost like a severe arthritis pain and can be treated as such. This pain does improve with time.

Breast cancer is the prototype of cancers that are dependent on hormones in women, analogous to prostate cancer in men. This is why some have suggested that shutting down the ovaries, the main source of estrogen, should be a mainstay approach in treating breast cancer. Another theorized advantage is that doing this might allow women to use drugs that could otherwise only be used in the postmenopausal state. Inducing women into menopause can be achieved by removing the ovaries surgically or by giving drugs like the LHRH injections that we mentioned earlier in our prostate cancer discussion. But sending women into immediate menopause brings up its own host of issues, both physical and emotional.

While beyond the scope of this text, it is noteworthy to mention that there are scenarios where women are placed on tamoxifen first and then switched to AIs or are placed on AIs alone from the get-go.

Duration of therapy could be a chapter by itself, so let me say that the field has evolved to recommend anywhere from 5 to 10 years of adjuvant hormonal therapy in women who have undergone surgery for early stage disease, with the idea that these hormonal therapies reduce the risk of recurrence. Remember that this is only given when there is evidence of estrogen receptor–positive or progesterone receptor–positive disease. These hormonal maneuvers are also used in disease that has spread as long as the receptors are considered positive.

Uterine cancer: Uterine cancer is another type of cancer that can be treated with hormones; the most common ones are progestins. A commonly used one is called medroxyprogesterone (Provera), which can be taken as a pill or an injection. The other one is megestrol (Megace), which can be consumed as pills or liquid.

There are other cancers that produce hormones or that use hormones as an essential part of their treatment. Adrenal cancers, for example, can produce excess hormonal products, and the treatment must control such excess production. Thyroid cancer requires replacing the thyroid hormone, which might be needed if the thyroid gland is removed as part of treating the cancer.

Regardless of the disease and of the hormonal therapy being used, it is essential to pay attention to side effects. Some of these that are often overlooked are anxiety, depression, and emotional changes. This is not surprising, since hormonal balance is being challenged in the body. I always spent enough time with my patients setting their expectations. Discussing sexual side effects is also important. These intimate topics are not always easy to address, and often patients don't bring them up. I view this as a responsibility of the treating doctor to put it out there and start the conversation.

Please talk to your doctor about what to expect.

Take-Home Points

- Some cancers depend on hormones to grow, multiply, and spread.

- Treating these cancers with hormonal therapies might help control the cancer (when we can't cure it) or cure it (as part of a larger regimen).

  ○ When hormonal therapy is given before the definitive treatment of the cancer, it is labeled as neoadjuvant therapy.

  ○ When hormonal therapy is given after the definitive treatment of the cancer, it is labeled as adjuvant therapy.

- Breast cancers and prostate cancers are the prototypes of cancers that are hormonally dependent, with the former depending on estrogen and the latter on testosterone.

- Patients and doctors must be vigilant about the side effects of hormonal therapies and take measures to either prevent them when possible or mitigate them when they occur.

CHAPTER 13

Treating the Cancer: Targeted Therapy

If you can't explain it simply,
you don't understand it well enough.

—*Albert Einstein*

ACCORDING TO THE EDITORIAL BOARD of www.cancer.net, targeted therapy is a type of cancer treatment that uses drugs to target specific genes and proteins that help cancer cells survive and grow. Targeted therapy can affect the tissue environment that cancer cells grow in, or it can target cells related to cancer growth, like blood vessel cells.

It was at the American Society of Hematology meeting in Orlando where I took my seat at the plenary session anticipating the presentation of Dr. Bertrand Coiffier from France on treating patients with diffuse large B-cell lymphoma, a form of aggressive non-Hodgkin lymphoma. For several decades, this disease had been treated with a chemotherapy regimen called CHOP (each letter denotes a chemotherapy drug), and no regimen had been shown to improve on the outcomes of that CHOP program. Until 2001.

Plenary presentations at medical society meetings are the most prestigious ones, usually reserved for presentations that share significant treatment implications that could change the standard of care, or basic science data that highlight the knowledge of a disease and its biology.

That day, the room was packed. I was completing my fellowship at Northwestern and was always thankful that the institution agreed to bear the cost of my travel. Dr. Coiffier showed that adding a drug called rituximab (Rituxan) to the CHOP program made patients live longer and reduced the risk of the lymphoma coming back. This was a major advance. This study was specifically designed for patients between the ages of 60 and 80, but other studies were being done in various age groups.

Rituximab is an antibody against CD20. Think of CD20 as a small protein on the surface of the cancer cell, and in lymphoma, there is a lot of that CD20. Rituximab is the bullet that targets that protein. The idea is that when the bullet reaches its target, the cell will die. Because the target exists on the cancer cell and not on the normal healthy cell, only cancer cells die, while normal cells survive. It can't get any more targeted than that.

It wasn't the first time that rituximab had made headline news. In fact, it had been approved by the FDA to treat a different form of non-Hodgkin lymphoma a few years back (November 1997, to be exact) and was being studied in all kinds of non-Hodgkin lymphoma, but that trial made news like no other because observers, doctors, and researchers knew that treating this disease had forever changed. The results of that study were eventually published in the most prestigious medical journal in the world, the *New England Journal of Medicine*.

Some may argue that rituximab was one of the first real targeted therapies showing a benefit to patients with cancer, but occasionally I try to play devil's advocate and challenge students with the question: Why not call any chemotherapy a targeted therapy? Chemotherapies, as you have learned, target the DNA strands and prevent cell growth; isn't that targeted? The difference is simple. Chemotherapy does not differentiate between normal and cancer cells, and side effects from chemotherapy emerge because of that. When normal cells are damaged, side effects occur, and patients can experience problems that we all want to avoid. With targeted therapy, the goal is to target only the cancer cells and spare the normal ones, which mitigates many side effects. This is what rituximab did. Certainly, there are other side effects that patients can experience from these targeted agents simply from the infusion itself, or allergic reactions and fatigue. With rituximab, as an example, some patients develop lower immunity since the drug targets B cells, which are essential to fight infections. But on balance, side effects from these targeted therapies are less severe than those from the traditional chemotherapies.

Around the time of Dr. Coiffier's plenary presentation, research was accelerating across all tumor types to find targeted therapies. The idea was attractive, and it resonated well with patients and with funding sources supporting clinical research. In breast cancer, researchers discovered a gene called *HER-2*, which leads the cells in the body to form receptors on their surfaces, making them divide and grow further; this gene was present in almost one quarter of breast cancers. Trastuzumab (Herceptin) is a breast cancer drug developed by Genentech, a biotech company located in South San Francisco, in collaboration with many academics. It targets these receptors and blocks the signal that leads to cell growth. At the time, in the late 1990s, it was known that breast cancers that had too much of this *HER-2* gene could have too many of these receptors and that their growth was dependent on the generated signal. Trastuzumab stopped those signals by attaching to the *HER-2* receptors on the surface of the breast cancer cells, and its discovery and activity revolutionized how breast cancer was treated forever.

Both trastuzumab and rituximab are examples of targeted therapies that belong to a class of drugs called *monoclonal antibodies*, but there are other classes of targeted agents that I will discuss later.

When I walked into the exam room one day, my new patient was immersed in reading what looked like a scientific article. He had prostate cancer that was requiring hormonal therapy. The year was 2002, and at the time, all that we could do for prostate cancers that had spread to other areas was to deprive the body of testosterone.

> *Patient:* I keep hearing about targeted therapies and how doctors can now target the cancers and kill these cancer cells.
>
> *CN:* This is absolutely true for some cancers, but not all. As you know, not all cancers are created equal, and the key is to know if a particular cancer has a target, and whether that target has a drug against it.
>
> *Patient:* So, there is no such thing for prostate cancer?
>
> *CN:* Not now, but lots of work is being done for that. For now, we use hormonal therapy, and hopefully that works for a long time.
>
> *Patient:* But there was this ad on the cover of *Time* magazine about some magic pill.
>
> *CN:* Yes; that pill works against a form of leukemia called CML [chronic myeloid leukemia]. It is not a pill against prostate cancer.

This kind of conversation occurs all over oncology clinics in America. Part of this difficulty is understanding that not all cancers are the same and that having a drug against a particular cancer does not mean that this drug works against other cancers. The prostate cancer conversation would be different today, as there are several targeted drugs available against this disease.

My patient's description of the *Time* magazine cover took me back to 1999, when I helped in a trial for chronic myelogenous leukemia (CML) using a drug labeled STI-571. I vividly remember how we would all be surprised with the amazing responses that we observed in patients enrolled in this trial. What was unique about this drug is that it was given orally. STI-571 eventually became known as imatinib mesylate, or Gleevec. The drug inhibits enzymes in the body that we normally call *tyrosine kinases*, which are involved in cell function and growth. The idea is that blocking these enzymes should stop cancer cells from growing, especially if they depend on these kinases to function.

It is impossible to write about targeted therapy and bring up the topic of CML without mentioning Dr. Janet Rowley, a pioneer scientist and geneticist who spent her career at the University of Chicago. I had always admired Dr. Rowley from afar but never met her until I joined the faculty of the University of Chicago in 2013. I had a few encounters with her when she visited the cancer center as a patient; she was humble, gracious with her time, and always grateful for the care she received. She ultimately died from ovarian cancer on December 17, 2013, at the age of 88. Dr. Rowley is credited as being the first scientist who identified chromosomal translocation as causing leukemias and other cancers. Translocations are events in which one piece from one chromosome can move to another chromosome while the latter chromosome loses a piece of its genetic material to the first chromosome. These exchanges in genetic material between two chromosomes can increase production of some proteins that play a major role in cell growth and cancer evolution. One example is the Philadelphia chromosome, which was originally discovered in the city that bears its name by Peter Nowell and David Hungerford in 1960. These two scientists found out that the Philadelphia chromosome, which refers to the shortened arm of chromosome 22, is present in cells of CML patients, but it wasn't clear how this short genetic material was developed until Dr. Rowley's seminal work demonstrated that this chromosome resulted from a reciprocal translocation of parts of chromosomes 9 and 22. Because of this exchange, an oncogene on chromosome 9 called the *c-abl* gets closer to a *bcr* gene on chromosome 22. This proximity produces a protein that plays a major role in transforming the white blood cells into cancerous cells, leading to the disease called CML. Nowell and Hungerford described the presence of this translocation in CML, but in 1973, Janet Rowley published her observations in the prestigious medical journal *Nature*, describing nine CML patients who all bore this translocation. Rowley and collaborators were able to further show that other types of leukemias can have chromosomal translocations and genetic material exchange, and that these exchanges are essential in how these forms of blood cancers were developing and growing. In fact, she is credited with discovering that the translocation of chromosomes 15 and 17 leads to a disease called *acute promyelocytic leukemia*, a type of leukemia that is cured in most patients as a result of this discovery, since therapies were designed to target the protein that is generated from this translocation. Dr. Rowley received numerous awards for these discoveries, including the National Medal of Science, the Presidential Medal of Freedom, and the lifetime achievement award by the American Association for Cancer Research, among many others. She had 14 honorary doctorates, including those from Oxford, Harvard, and Yale. I do not know why she never won the Nobel Prize, but in my opinion, she deserves to win a few Nobels.

It is fair to say that without this pioneering work done in the sixties and seventies, patients never would have had access to this drug depicted on the *Time* magazine cover, which transformed their lives positively forever.

As the name implies, targeted therapies are therapies designed against targets found in cancer cells. Research accelerated in the past 20 years to identify such targets; manufacturers of cancer drugs have also accelerated their research and development efforts to find drugs that can be effective against these targets. An ideal target would be a protein that is present in cancer cells but not in healthy cells; the designed therapies can turn off the signals that lead to cancer cell growth. Not all cancers have targets, however, and not all targets have drugs that work against them.

It is useful to think about targeted therapy in categories:

- **Monoclonal antibodies**: Rituximab and trastuzumab, the examples I gave earlier, are monoclonal antibodies. These are proteins that attach to targets found on the cancer cells. Side effects vary among people, but flu-like symptoms are not unusual. Some patients have allergic reactions that can vary in severity; others experience fluctuations in their blood pressure and cardiac side effects. I have always told my patients that I prefer not to list every single adverse event on a piece of paper because they won't call me asking for help unless they experience those exact side effects, and that specificity takes away from the nuances of how we differ as human beings. I have, however, always shared with them the top ones I have observed in patients similar to them. Some monoclonal antibodies are considered a form of immunotherapy, and these will be discussed in chapter 14.

- **Antibody drug conjugates (ADCs)**: Often, this is a monoclonal antibody that is coupled with another anticancer drug (usually some form of chemotherapy that can break the cell DNA).

As the antibody attaches to the target on the cancer cell, the antibody with its linked drug gets internalized and the cancer cell dies.

- **Small molecules**: As the name implies, these drugs are small, allowing them to enter the cancer cell and exert their activity within. These molecules are often given by mouth and can target the cancer cell using different mechanisms of action, but commonly, they inhibit one or two pathways within the cancer cells that lead to their growth. By doing so, cancer cells can stop multiplying and growing.

- **Antiangionenesis**: These can be monoclonal antibodies or small molecules. To step back, the word "angiogenesis" means forming blood vessels. These formations can occur in health and in disease, including cancer. In order for tumors to grow, they need nutrients to keep them growing, and these can be supplied via blood vessels around the tumor. Also, the tumor itself can generate signals that lead to forming more blood vessels, so we end up in a vicious cycle. You recall also that cancers spread to distant organs through blood vessels that carry the cancer cells to different locations, so these blood vessels are integral in many types of cancer. Drugs that are classified as angiogenesis inhibitors block the blood vessel growth and in turn can "starve" the tumor from what it needs. The way these drugs work is by interfering in the pathways that lead to blood vessel growth. Some of these drugs are monoclonal antibodies, so they are designed to specifically target a protein called *vascular endothelial growth factor* (VEGF), which is needed to form these blood vessels. Other drugs can bind to the receptor that VEGF was supposed to get attached to, preventing this unity between VEGF and its receptor. There are some drugs that affect blood vessel growth but also have ways to enhance the immune system to fight cancer cells.

Some antiangiogenesis drugs are given intravenously (bevaci-zumab [Avastin] as an example), while others are given orally (axitinib, cabozantinib, and others). These drugs can be very ef-fective, but caution is needed to minimize side effects. I recall having to memorize a lot about managing high blood pressure when bevacizumab came to market because hypertension is one of its most well-known side effects. This is not surprising as blood pressure elevation can occur from more blood vessel for-mation and constriction. Other side effects include delayed wound healing, so sometimes we have to postpone minor sur-geries in patients who receive these agents, including dental procedures. Bleeding and clotting can both occur when using these drugs, but I think the most serious side effect that can be encountered is what we call *bowel perforation*. This is when a hole is formed in the intestines; it can require emergent surgery and cannot be delayed. When this occurs, patients experience severe abdominal pain that is not easily relieved.

Some stories stay with us forever. I recall being called to see a young woman around the age of 40 who was having difficulty breathing. Her CT scans showed changes in her lungs that were very suspicious. She had never smoked, but the radiologist told me that this pattern was more likely than not a form of disseminated lung cancer. The rest of her CT scans showed no disease outside the chest. Because she re-quired so much oxygen, and there was a fear that she might end up on a breathing machine, she was admitted to the intensive care unit, where we first met.

As you have learned, we must always get a tissue biopsy to decide what to do. There was no doubt in my mind that this was a form of cancer, but the exact type of cancer was still in question. A pulmon-ologist performed an urgent procedure to get tissue. I did have a backup plan of what I would do in case things got worse, but I was hoping that time stayed on my side until the diagnosis was certain.

The pathologist called and said it was non-small cell lung cancer. The year was 2005, and a drug called erlotinib had just been approved several months prior in patients with metastatic non-small cell lung cancer. At the time, mechanisms by which erlotinib (Tarceva) worked were not fully understood, but we knew from clinical trial data that patients who benefited the most were those who were of Asian descent, had adenocarcinoma cells under the microscope, were females, and had never smoked. My patient, who was in so much distress and could barely breathe, had all these factors. Erlotinib, as a drug, is considered a tyrosine kinase inhibitor, and it blocks a protein on the surface of cancer cells called *epidermal growth factor receptor*, or EGFR. By targeting the EGFR, it blocks tumor cells from growing. Originally, we knew that this drug worked if we could detect the presence of these receptors on the cancer cells, but later on we knew that erlotinib worked if there were specific mutations in these receptors. This was important as the decision to use it was no longer based on the four patient characteristics I mentioned above and the simple staining of the EGFR, but rather on a specific mutation that we had to detect, which could be present in smokers and in men, as an example.

I had started her on chemotherapy the minute I confirmed that she had lung cancer, hoping that this would improve her breathing. Once I was able to get her the erlotinib, I started her on that medication and stopped chemotherapy altogether. Within three weeks she was discharged from the hospital, requiring no oxygen. I could not believe my eyes when I saw her with her family in my office looking vibrant and optimistic. When she canceled her visit with me one day because she had a hair appointment, I knew that we were on the right path.

The story of how lung cancer has evolved is one of many stories that defined the success of targeted therapies. The disease was once classified into only two broad categories based on how the cells looked and stained under the microscope. Now, lung cancer is divided into many categories based on the mutation that leads to cancer growth. What is unique is the explosion of new therapies targeted against these mutations that have made a big difference in patients' lives. Examples of the success of targeted therapies across various cancers are beyond one chapter, but I know you got the gist and understand the success.

We still have a lot to do. First, not every cancer has a target, and not every target has a treatment against it. Even when there is a target and a treatment, the latter doesn't work all the time, and when it does, it does not work forever. But every step is hopefully heading in the right direction of making cancer a chronic disease managed like we manage high blood pressure or diabetes.

Take-Home Points

- Targeted therapies are various treatments that attack a target on the cancer cells, sparing the normal cells.

- There are various types, such as monoclonal antibodies, antibody drug conjugates, small molecules, and antiangionenesis.

- Not every cancer has a target with an available drug against it, and even then not all patients respond.

- Side effects of targeted therapies are generally milder than traditional chemotherapies. Some of these therapies are given intravenously, while others are delivered under the skin or orally.

CHAPTER 14

Treating the Cancer: Immunotherapy

If you want the present to be different
from the past, study the past.

—*Baruch Spinoza*

OUR BODY HAS MECHANISMS to protect us from outside invaders. When new substances enter our body, the guards in the immune system are alerted to shield us from these external intruders, which can be germs (bacteria, viruses, or other agents) or cancer cells. The job of the immune system is to recognize cells that belong to us and to identify cells that don't so that they are removed. The most important guarding cells we have are called *T cells*.

The theory is that in some circumstances the immune system is sleepy and is not doing its job. Think of this like sleepy guards of a bank or a security system that is broken, both scenarios that can lead to robberies. What needs to happen is either boosting, or waking up, the existing immune system and repairing it or creating a new system if the current one is completely dysfunctional.

Immunotherapy is a type of treatment that is focused on helping the immune system fight cancer cells. This is not simple, however, since cancer cells usually evolve from normal cells, making it challenging to recognize these cells as foreign. This is partly why cancer can evade the immune system and trick it to an extent. We just need to be smarter than these tricks.

Let's think this through. Why would the immune system not do its job? What are the possibilities? Maybe the cancer cells look like normal cells, or maybe they do look different, but the immune system is not strong enough to overcome their power. Maybe the cancer cells produce proteins or other substances that by themselves attack the immune system, which puts the immune system on the offense.

Bottom line—we need to find ways to make the immune system work in our favor. How do we do that?

- **Monoclonal antibodies**: Recall that we discussed these when we reviewed targeted therapy. These are medications that scientists make in the laboratory so that they can attack cancer cells. The antibodies are manufactured against proteins that are present on the cancer cells but not on normal cells. This way, we can minimize side effects because normal healthy cells are somewhat spared. The proteins present on the cancer cells are called *antigens*. Once the antibodies are given to patients, they circulate in the blood until they find the target they were designed to attach to—the antigens. Once attached, the immune system is stimulated, among other things, and this improves the drug's ability to destroy cancer cells. The most important part of this process is to identify the antigen that can be targeted. Sometimes an antigen cannot be identified, while other times we are unable to manufacture an antibody to an identified antigen. So, monoclonal antibodies are man-made proteins, meaning they are not natural or organic. Manufacturing them can be daunting;

sometimes it is done from mouse proteins, human proteins, or a combination when made from small parts of mouse proteins attached to human ones (we call these *chimeric proteins*).

Occasionally, these antibodies have something else attached to them so they act like a delivery system. One example is a type of drug called radioimmunoconjugates; these are antibodies with some form of radiation attached to them. They go to the antigen and deliver the radiation that eventually can kill the cancer cells (I mentioned this briefly in chapter 11). When chemotherapy is attached to the antibody, the chemotoxin gets internalized into the cancer cell to kill it. One of the first articles I ever wrote was on treating leukemia patients with a drug called Mylotarg (gemtuzumab ozogamicin), an antibody against CD33, which is the antigen on acute myeloid leukemia cells. The antibody is attached to a drug called calicheamicin or ozogamicin, which gets into the leukemia cell after the antibody attaches to the CD33 antigen. The antibodies that have nothing attached to them are labeled as "naked" antibodies, while all others are called "conjugated." The term *antibody drug conjugates* was born when scientists were able to add various drugs, such as chemotherapy, to the monoclonal antibodies, and nowadays, there are too many examples of these to list.

• **Bispecific monoclonal antibodies**: These interesting antibodies have gained popularity in the past five years or so after several new drugs belonging to this category were approved. As their name implies, these antibodies can bind to two proteins at the same time. One protein is the antigen on the cancer cell, and the other is a protein present on the T cells, so they get stimulated. By binding to these two proteins, these drugs essentially bring the T cells or the defender cells near the cancer cells, with the theory that this makes them more effective at killing the foreign cancer cells.

- **Checkpoint inhibitors:** Recall that T cells differentiate between normal cells and foreign cells, attacking the latter while sparing the former. It turns out that our body places "checkpoints" in front of the normal cells so they don't get attacked. Think of these as stop signs on the road. The cars (T cells here) must stop and in doing so, normal cells are left alone. The stop signs tell our immune system not to destroy the cells that belong to our body. Cancer cells play a few tricks on these stop signs, stealing them to trick the immune system into thinking they are like any normal cells. This in turn prevents the immune system from attacking these cancer cells. In essence, cancer cells hold on to these stop signs and pretend they are normal, so the immune system becomes helpless, unable to do much against them. Scientists have been working on developing drugs that get rid of these stop signs to push the immune system to start attacking the cancer cells. These drugs are what we call *checkpoint inhibitors*. Think of them as preventing the cancer from blocking the immune system. There are different types of checkpoints or stop signs, but the most important ones are PD1, PD-L1, CTLA-4, and LAG-3. Various drugs have been developed to target any of these checkpoints, and several of these drugs are approved for treating various cancers. What has become interesting is that some of these checkpoint inhibitors were approved regardless of where the tumor had originated. One of the most important things to monitor when using these drugs are autoimmune reactions, as these occur because the immune system starts making mistakes and identifies normal cells as foreign ones, subsequently attacking them. Some of these autoimmune reactions can be severe, such as inflammation of the colon, thyroid, and other organs, while occasionally, they can be mild. When targeting the checkpoint proteins, these drugs essentially get rid of one of our body's important safeguards, so our body might get in trouble. I always tell patients to communicate all side effects with their doctor, as some might be serious enough to stop the drug and start treatment with steroids or other drugs that ameliorate the side effects. Of course, there are other side effects that might occur, such as fatigue, nausea, diarrhea, and infusion-related adverse events.

It's interesting to mention that the activity of the checkpoint inhibitors targeting PD1 or PD-L1 is sometimes linked to the percentage of tumor cells expressing these proteins on their surface. The expression of these proteins is determined by something called *tumor proportion score*, or TPS, which is the percentage of viable tumor cells showing partial or complete staining of any intensity on the membrane. If the TPS is greater than or equal to 1%, then the expression is positive, but if it exceeds 50%, then we call that expression high. We calculate TPS by counting the number of PD-L1–positive tumor cells and dividing that by the total number of all tumor cells, then multiply the results by 100. Sometimes, pathologists look at the composite positive score (CPS), the ratio of tumor cells expressing PD-L1 in addition to immune cells that could express these proteins. From a patient perspective, what you need to ask your doctor is if your tumor cells are PD1 or PD-L1. It is reassuring to know that these are now tested routinely in every pathology lab and in almost all cancer specimens.

- **Cancer vaccines:** The minute we hear the word "vaccine," we assume that we are talking about preventing or mitigating an illness. In oncology, cancer vaccines have a different meaning.

I was at Advocate Lutheran General Hospital when I was approached by a small Seattle-based company to consider opening a study they were sponsoring for patients with metastatic prostate cancer. Dendreon was developing a vaccine to treat some form of prostate cancer. I recall many patients would see me because they assumed they would get a shot that would prevent the development of future prostate cancer, and I would spend time explaining that that was not the case. This does not suggest that there aren't vaccines that might prevent certain cancers, but these generally prevent viruses known to cause cancers from being transmitted.

○ *Vaccines that treat cancer*: I have always thought that we should name these something else to avoid confusion, but I doubt that will ever happen. So, think of cancer vaccines as a way to strengthen patients' immune systems to fight cancer. Like I said before, cancer cells have proteins, or antigens, that are not generally present on normal cells. These vaccines train the immune system to recognize these antigens as "bad ones" so that cancer cells are destroyed. The vaccine I was involved in is called Provenge (Sipuleucel-T). Basically, it was manufactured by taking immune cells called *dendritic cells* from the patient. These are cells that can boost the immune system by showing antigens on their surface to other cells of the immune system; this is why we call these dendritic cells *antigen-presenting cells*, or APCs. To make the Provenge vaccine, these APCs are taken from the patient and exposed to a protein or an antigen that is specific to prostate cancer, called prostatic acid phosphatase (PAP). Once the APCs are infused back into the patient, they attack prostate cancer cells that have PAPs. With Provenge, the "vaccine" is given by vein three times, each dose two weeks apart. This vaccine is made from the patient's own immune cells, so we call it an "autologous" vaccine, but there are others that are manufactured differently with the same general concept. Occasionally, scientists can make these vaccines from the patient's own tumor or cancer cells, so when administered, they exert activity against these cells. There are also ways we can infect malignant (cancerous) cells with viruses that kill the cancer cells; these viruses are called *oncolytic viruses*, and they don't damage normal cells. There is one such vaccine that is approved by the FDA, called T-VEC, which is usually injected directly into the tumor. Generally, it has been used in melanoma.

o *Vaccines that prevent cancer*: Certain strains of HPV have been associated with increased risk of cervical cancer, among other cancers. Vaccinating children and young adults against HPV protects against these cancers. Another example is the hepatitis B virus, which can lead to liver cancer in certain situations, and therefore vaccinating against it is recommended.

When it comes to side effects of these vaccine-type therapies, one can expect mild flu-like symptoms such as fevers, chills, weakness, fatigue, headaches, and muscle aches. Generally, these are well tolerated, although I have seen variations in their severity. Sometimes, patients encounter reactions around the injection site or unexpected allergies to ingredients that compose these vaccines. These vaccines are sometimes combined with additional proteins that boost their immune response, and patients can react to these "adjuvant" compounds as well. Overall, cancer vaccines are well tolerated, but I admit that I am on the fence as to how robust their activity is across various tumor types. In my opinion, the jury remains out on how best to use vaccine treatments and how best to optimize them.

• **Nonspecific immunotherapy**: These agents can help stimulate the immune system but are not specific to a tumor or to a patient (hence their name). Examples include drugs called interferons, interleukins, and BCG (Bacillus Calmette-Guerin). It turns out that some cancers may be more responsive to these type of therapies (melanoma and kidney cancers), while others are not.

Scientists continue to explore how best to make more patients benefit from immunotherapy.

Back when I was a fellow, one of the most important questions in melanoma was whether we should give patients interferon after the tumor had been removed. I recall seeing a woman in her late thirties who had a large leg melanoma, and the entire conversation we had was whether she should get interferon. Fast-forward to today, and virtually no patient with melanoma receives interferon anymore.

Another example is the change we have seen with kidney cancer. Patients with kidney cancer used to be admitted to the hospital to receive high doses of interleukin 2. They would be so sick in the ICU, barely able to breathe for the hope that less than 5% of them might go into remission. Today, virtually no patient with kidney cancer receives interleukin.

- **Immunomodulators**: These are drugs that we think enhance the immune system somehow. There are so many of them nowadays. In 1999, a paper in the *New England Journal of Medicine* showed that thalidomide worked in patients with multiple myeloma, a form of a bone marrow cancer. Thalidomide had been banned in the 1970s because it had caused limb deformities when taken as a sleeping aid by pregnant women. Fast-forward a few decades after that ban, and it became an active drug against one of the most fatal cancers. I can't recall how many papers were written trying to explain how thalidomide works, but some proposed that it manipulates the immune system and thereby helps it fight cancer. It turns out that thalidomide also has antiangiogenesis properties and helps the body release interleukins to fight cancer cells. After its development, scientists manufactured more powerful immune modulators that are more effective and less toxic. I still think we don't have a full grasp on how these drugs work, but we know that they do, and they have certainly saved many lives over the years.

What is very interesting about immunotherapy is deciding how we know if it works.

I had a patient on a clinical trial of a checkpoint inhibitor; he was supposed to have a CT scan every two months to assess his response. The first scan showed that some of the lesions I was monitoring were enlarging. I walked into the exam room and was pleasantly surprised that he looked well. I was expecting that he would be feeling worse considering that his scans were not improving. His blood work was also OK.

CN: How do you feel?

Patient: I feel well, actually; my cough is much better, and I am sleeping better at night.

CN: So, compared with the last time we saw each other, you're feeling better.

Patient: At least not worse; maybe slightly better, but not worse.

CN: Let's go over your scans. The areas we have been monitoring in the lungs appear larger than in the last scan, but you look much better clinically. Even your blood work and exam are OK and have not changed.

Patient: What do you suggest we do?

CN: Well, you're on a clinical trial. I need to call the medical monitor since technically we need to stop the treatment, but I don't think we should.

The trial was sponsored by the manufacturer of the drug being used. Companies usually assign medical monitors to every study of theirs to ensure the conduct of the trial is appropriate and to answer questions from treating physicians like me. I told my patient that I would get back to him within 24 hours as I needed to discuss his case with the monitor.

When I reached the medical monitor, he informed me that the company had been getting similar reports from various treating physicians who had patients on their trial, and they were going to amend the study to allow treatment to continue as long as patients were feeling well.

This made sense to me. I have always told patients, friends, and family that we don't treat "scans" or "labs"; we treat patients. We cannot throw our clinical judgment out the window and only treat what we see on imaging studies.

I called the patient. "Good news; we will stay on the drug. Looks like other patients are experiencing the same," I said. He thanked me and commented that he believed the drug was working regardless of what the scans showed.

It turns out that patients on these kinds of immunotherapy might experience inflammation and some other reactions that artificially suggest the disease is getting worse based on the scans, but that's not the case. Scientifically, we started calling this phenomenon *pseudoprogression*, and eventually the scientific community embraced it and even developed criteria specific to immunotherapy to help physicians decide whether patients are benefiting.

So, for these immunotherapies, we look at the big picture and not only the size of the areas we are monitoring. Had we not adjusted our response assessment, many of these treatments would not have seen the light, and many patients would not have been helped.

So many questions remain when it comes to immunotherapy. Why do some patients respond while others don't? Can we do more to optimize the response and outcomes of patients receiving immunotherapy? Should we use immunotherapy alone, or is it better to add it to other agents? Can we predict who might respond so that we don't give the treatment unless there is a high likelihood of responding? How can we reduce the side effects? Does developing side effects indicate that treatment is working?

I am hoping that continued research will lead us to answer some of these important questions.

Take-Home Points

- Immunotherapy is a treatment approach that makes our own immune system attack cancer cells and identify them as foreign cells.

- Different types of immunotherapies exist, but notable advances have been in checkpoint inhibitors and cancer vaccines.

- The type of side effects are different with these; we must pay extra attention to severe autoimmune adverse events, which might require stopping therapy and administering steroids.

- Sometimes, imaging studies might show the tumor is growing while the patient is in fact responding to treatment. We call this pseudo-progression, and your doctor will determine next steps—often, patients are continued on therapy and are monitored.

CHAPTER 15

Bone Marrow Transplantation and Cellular Therapy

There is no innovation and creativity
without failure. Period.

—*Brené Brown*

ONE OF THE FIRST ROTATIONS I did when I started my residency at Loyola University in Chicago was in the bone marrow transplant (BMT) unit. I probably should have known more about BMT, but having done my medical school in Syria, I had little exposure to that technology, so my understanding of the concept was minimal. Still, I was looking forward to learning. As a refresher, think of the bone marrow as the factory that produces all the functioning cells in our blood system. We need red cells to carry oxygen throughout the body, white cells to fend off infections, and platelets to protect us from bleeding; these cells are generated in the bone marrow from their baby cells, mature, and then get out of the factory to circulate throughout, doing what they were made to do. As the BMT name implies, I had assumed that we would replace the diseased and sick bone marrow with a new marrow and to do that, we needed surgery. I was partially correct, but way off on how this is done.

There was no surgery to replace a marrow with another, but I was once asked to scrub because I was to assist my attendings who were collecting bone marrow from the sister of a patient with leukemia. Extracting the healthy bone marrow from the sister was to be done in the operating room under general anesthesia. This procedure is done just like we do bone marrow aspirates and biopsies at the bedside, but because we were extracting so much marrow, we were essentially subjecting the sister to numerous aspirates within a short period of time, which would be very painful—thus the general anesthesia and the need for the operating room. The year was 1995, and much has changed since then.

It's probably a good idea to start by understanding the different kinds of BMT:

- **Syngenic**: This is when we take the bone marrow of an identical twin and give it to the diseased twin; the blood types will match exactly. These are considered the least complicated, and the recipient is unlikely to reject the "new" marrow as it comes from their identical twin.

- **Allogeneic**: This is from a donor matched to the patient, generally a sibling. It also can be from an unrelated matched donor. To check whether a potential donor is a match, a blood test is done to evaluate the human leukocyte antigens (HLAs), which are antigens (think proteins on the surface of the cells) that we would prefer to be matched between patients and their donors. There are 12 HLAs, and a full match happens when all these antigens are similar between the donor and the recipient.

- **Haploidentical**: It is not always easy to find a match for a patient, which happens more often in underrepresented minorities. This is important as children and parents of patients are all half-matched. Half-identical donors can donate their marrows with almost a similar favorable outcome to fully matched donors when transplant is done in specialized centers. This provides an immediate source for a donor when needed. Because of the improved ability to conduct these transplants, almost any patient needing an allogeneic transplant can now get one.

- **Umbilical cord**: Partially matched umbilical cord blood has become a source of BMT. This is used more in the pediatric population but is gaining popularity in adults.

- **Autologous**: This means that the source of the marrow is the patient.

I never liked surgery, so when I was asked to assist in collecting bone marrow cells in the operating room, I felt out of place, but I had to do what my superiors asked me to do. The first time I assisted with that, the donor was the sister of a patient with leukemia. We used the bone marrow biopsy needles and kept poking the hip bones for two hours to aspirate blood from inside the marrow. That collected marrow would be preserved so that we could eventually give it to the patient who needed it.

My attending explained, "We are collecting her stem cells from the healthy bone marrow. These particular stem cells are immature cells that grow into all blood cells in our body: white cells, red cells, and platelets." He explained how these stem cells could divide and multiply to make newer stem cells. He also explained that the bone marrow is the space where most of the stem cells exist, and because there are more marrow cells in larger bones, we collect the bone marrow from the hip bones.

Today, we can collect good stem cells from the blood. Since these stem cells are generated in the bone marrow and then exit that space into the blood, we can collect them from the blood through the vein versus putting these large bore needles in the hip bones. This understanding led to the gradual shifting of the procedure's name from BMT to stem cell transplant, or SCT. Because SCT is done through the hematologic system, the process is now commonly referred to as hematopoietic stem cell transplantation (HSCT). A BMT takes the stem cells from your bone marrow. An SCT takes the stem cells from your bone marrow or your bloodstream.

Because these stem cells that are usually found in the bone marrow are located in the peripheral blood (the blood that circulates in our veins and arteries), we started collecting them without needing a surgical procedure and general anesthesia, regardless of whether we are collecting them from the patient (in autologous scenarios) or the donor (in allogeneic situations). To collect them, the donor is given injections of white blood cell growth factor (the same injections we sometimes use after chemotherapy to prevent white blood cells from dropping to dangerously low levels); these injections are called filgrastim (Neupogen). Usually, the donor receives these injections daily for about five days because this helps mobilize the stem cells from the marrow so that we can collect them. The stem cells are collected through the veins through a procedure called *apheresis*. The blood is removed from one arm through a vein and passed to a machine that checks and collects these blood-forming cells, and the remaining blood is returned to the patient. Think of this as the donor giving blood in an outpatient procedure. Generally, this is done once, but there are situations when the donor needs two sessions to collect enough stem cells to be later infused into the patient's blood system. Aside from muscle and bone aches, this procedure is well tolerated, but fatigue can last up to seven days post-procedure.

Let's discuss each type of transplant in more detail.

Autologous Transplant

Now that we don't use the bone marrow, autologous transplant is better labeled autologous stem cell transplant. The concept is that we take the stem cells from the patient, but logically we should do that after the patient is in remission so that the stem cells are clear of any possible cancer. Therefore, patients must receive chemotherapy before collecting these stem cells, with the idea that this chemotherapy clears the cancer cells that we normally see on imaging studies. We know, however, that this is not usually enough to eradicate the cancer, so as part of the plan, we further treat the cancer cells with high doses of additional chemotherapy. These high doses of chemotherapy are what we call a *conditioning regimen*. When we give chemotherapy at such high doses, the healthy stem cells and the immune system of the patients are damaged, and this is exactly why we collect the stem cells before we give these high doses of chemotherapy so that we can give them back to the patients to restore their immune system. In essence, we give chemotherapy to eradicate whatever we can see on scans, PET, or other imaging studies; then, we collect the stem cells as mentioned above. This is followed by the conditioning regimen, which kills any cancer cells that we might have missed, as imaging can't ever be sensitive enough to pick up everything. Because these higher doses are damaging to normal healthy cells in addition to cancer cells, we infuse back into the patient's bloodstream the previously collected stem cells. A better term, therefore, is stem cell rescue, as we are rescuing the damaged immune system. Many contend that labeling this procedure as stem cell transplantation is inaccurate, and we should change it to "high-dose chemotherapy and stem cell rescue."

To simplify, think of autologous transplant as a stepwise approach:

1. Giving chemotherapy to put the patient in the most remission possible.

2. Collecting the stem cells via the apheresis procedure, as described above.

3. Giving high doses of chemotherapy (sometimes radiation) over four or five days to really clean the bloodstream of any remaining cancer cells, but this usually damages healthy normal cells.

4. Infusing the stem cells back. This is reinfusion day; it's like getting a blood transfusion, and it is done in 30–45 minutes or so. Usually, patients get one infusion, but it can be more than one. This transplant day is called day 0. When patients are on high doses of chemotherapy, they are monitored carefully for any infections and are on prophylactic antibiotics (antibiotics that we give in the absence of an active infection with the hopes that they can prevent an infection from happening) to minimize such risks. They are also on antiviral and sometimes antifungal medications and other drugs that attempt to reduce side effects.

5. Wait and see. This is the recovery period where we wait for these stem cells to do their job: populate the bloodstream with white blood cells. Patients often require blood transfusions and platelets until the stem cells start functioning and the patient's marrow starts doing its job of making new, healthy blood cells. The time it takes until the infused stem cells start working varies, ranging from 7 to 14 days. Infrequently, I had patients who took longer. Once the white cells start climbing up, the risk of infection goes down substantially.

Allogeneic Transplant

With allogeneic transplant, the stem cells are taken from a donor, not the patient. Ideally, we prefer that the patient has as little cancer as possible before they get the stem cells from the donor, which is why patients also receive chemotherapy before transplant to get them into the best remission possible. This allogeneic procedure, when successful, provides the patient with an entirely new immune system and new stem cells from a wholly healthy donor, so even if some cancer is left behind after the chemotherapy, this new immune system could and might attack the remaining cancer cells. We call this the *graft versus tumor effect*. The graft is the new stem cells, and the tumor is the cancer we are treating. Patients still undergo very high doses of chemotherapy and radiation (conditioning regimen), which wipe out potentially remaining cancer cells as well as healthy cells. We then must rescue the patient by reinfusing the stem cells that we had already collected from the donor. The benefit of this kind of transplant is obvious.

In autologous stem cell transplant, there is always the risk that the reinfused cells might contain some cancer cells that we don't see, since the source of the stem cells is the patient who had the cancer; we call this *contamination*. In allogeneic transplant, there cannot be any contamination, as the stem cells come from a healthy donor. Indeed, the graft versus cancer effect can be essential in treating the underlying problem. The disadvantage is that we cannot always find that perfect donor. Still, that disadvantage is less today than when I did my residency, as technology has allowed us to give stem cells from unrelated donors or donors that are not an ideal match. Let's look at this stepwise approach to allogeneic transplant.

1. **Identify the donor.** Once a decision is made that an allogeneic transplant is indicated, the most crucial step is finding the donor. To find a match, we perform HLA typing, where the doctors check the HLA type and try to find a match. Doctors start by looking at the patient's siblings if applicable and at the bone marrow registry, a list of names and HLA types of donors who are willing to give their healthy stem cells when called upon.

2. **Collect the stem cells from the donor using the apheresis procedure.** The donor, as we discussed, will get these shots that allow us to collect their stem cells from their vein. As I mentioned, when I did residency, we had to do that in the OR from the hip bones, and that procedure, called *bone marrow harvest*, is rarely if ever done now.

3. **Administer chemotherapy.** High doses of chemotherapy with or without radiation are given to the patient while hospitalized. These are done over five days or so.

4. **Infuse the stem cells.** Day 0 is when the patient receives the stem cells from the donor, just like getting a blood transfusion. This takes 30–45 minutes and generally is one infusion.

5. **Recover.** Again, we wait until stem cells start doing their job with all prophylactic measures in place.

Mini-allogeneic Transplant (Nonmyeloablative)

Mini-allogeneic transplant means the patient receives "less" intense chemotherapy than the traditional conditioning program. The idea is to benefit from the transplant while minimizing possible side effects, which are more likely with higher doses of traditional conditioning chemotherapy. This type of transplant is generally offered to older patients whose doctors believe they cannot tolerate the higher doses.

Umbilical Cord Transplant

It turns out that umbilical cords, usually disposed of in the past as an unnecessary by-product of birth, contain a wealth of stem cells, which can be used for a variety of purposes, including in patients who need stem cell transplants. Thousands of cord transplants have been done worldwide as the process of collecting umbilical stem cells is simple; it takes less than 10 minutes, but the cords must be donated, and parents have to agree. Parents who want to donate should discuss this with their healthcare team before delivery. The hospital where delivery takes place coordinates with the cord blood bank ahead of time; parents can also contact the National Marrow Donor Program (NMDP) to get more guidance. Some families choose to donate for their potential future usage; this requires private storage, which will cost money, but if the donation is for whomever needs to use it (placed in what we call *public storage*), then the harvesting is free. Here is the basic process:

1. After the birth of a baby, the doctor cuts and clamps the cord.

2. The doctor collects 3–5 ounces of blood from the umbilical cord and placenta.

3. After donation, the cord blood will be HLA typed and placed in the donor registry.

4. Cord blood is stored in a special freezer until there is a match with a patient in need.

5. The process then follows the allogeneic process that I described above.

Haplo-mismatched Transplant

A haplo-mismatched transplant indicates a mismatch in the donor to recipient where we know there is a 50% match for sure, but the rest may not be. The source of the stem cells here is one of the parents or a child giving the stem cells to a parent. Regardless, it would be best if we thought of this as a transplant from a relative who is not a complete match to the patient. This has been used more lately as finding stem cells that patients need remains the most critical part of this process, and without them, patients can't be helped. Experienced transplant centers can do these transplants with excellent results, even though the match is less than perfect.

Haplo-cord Transplant

In a haplo-cord transplant, the source of the stem cells is dual: from an umbilical cord plus a haplo-donor. There are highly specialized centers that do these and various situations that might lead your doctor to recommend this kind of transplant.

I recall seeing her with her brother when I was rotating through the transplant clinic while doing my fellowship. She was 43 and had undergone SCT from her brother about a year before this visit. Her skin had what looked to me like scars from a healing rash that occupied most of her thin-framed and frail body. She was quiet and barely spoke, but she had a faint and friendly smile that left an impression on me almost 25 years after we met. As is customary in academic centers, I was to see her first and then describe my observations to my attending physician.

I checked her blood work, which was perfect. Her exam was regular, aside from the skin findings I described. I tried to have a light conversation with her and be reassuring, but she wasn't too conversational. In her prior chart notes, this particular issue wasn't highlighted much, but one message suggested that she had mild depression. Her brother confirmed that she had little interest in getting out of the house and being with friends.

I was taken aback by the visit. On the one hand, I was elated at how well she was doing. The cancer was gone; she was in remission; she was alive. On the other hand, she was sad, and I did not get the sense that she cared for being around.

I told my attending as such. He had cared for her for almost five years since she had been initially diagnosed with chronic myeloid leukemia. After various treatment rounds, her medical team decided to proceed with an allogeneic transplant as her brother was a complete match. At the time, this was the only therapy that could cure her. My attending shared how vibrant, outgoing, and social she used to be, but that had changed. He attributed her psychological state to the transplant; despite visits to the psychologist, no significant improvement was observed. We spent more time with her and her brother and scheduled her to see us back in three months.

I saw this patient throughout my fellowship. She died during my third year of training while in complete remission from her leukemia. She succumbed to infections that could not be cleared and were generated from her skin ulcers and scars that developed as a complication from her transplant. I knew she died depressed and could only imagine how miserable those past few years were for her and her family.

To this day, I think of that patient. She taught me that complications can sometimes be worse than the treatment itself. Ultimately, what matters the most is that our patients live longer and better. She did live longer, but not better. Did we help her? I don't know; it's impossible to tell, but this encounter taught me to put everything in perspective. While doctors and clinical trials focus on extending patient lives, we must recognize that many patients forgo extending their life span if this means jeopardizing their quality of life. It is essential to engage patients in these discussions, and frequently nowadays, patients have become involved in the design of large clinical trials so that their voice and values are heard and integrated. What we learn in medicine is that what matters to some patients might not be relevant to others, and each patient might represent a case series of one.

It's important to discuss the complications of these treatments and how best to counter them.

Complications of Autologous Transplant

- **Traditional side effects from the high-dose chemotherapy used before infusing the stem cells (a conditioning program).** These side effects depend on the type of chemo used; however, these high doses are destined to cause hair loss, infertility, nausea, vomiting, diarrhea, mouth sores (or what we call mucositis), and other toxicities. We have grown to know exactly what to expect when using these conditioning programs, so we usually prepare to counter potential side effects. Almost all of these side effects are reversible except infertility. In that case, doctors might recommend sperm banking or egg harvesting ahead of these treatments. The transplant team will provide information describing what to expect, but patients must ask the doctors, nurses, pharmacists, and everyone on the team about the type of remedies available.

- **Nontraditional side effects.** High-dose chemotherapy can lead to a liver disease called *veno-occlusive disease*, or VOD. It is severe and can cause significant problems. Doctors might prescribe prophylactic medicines to prevent it. Essentially, the vessels in the liver get damaged, and patients can become jaundiced with an enlarged liver. I saw this more with the allogeneic transplant than the autologous transplant. I also put here the side effects that are very specific for some chemo drugs. In other words, all chemotherapies cause fatigue, but not all make patients prone to seizures. These rare but possible side effects must be discussed, and more importantly, measures must be taken to minimize their likelihood.

- **Infections.** The chemotherapy will bring down white blood cell counts, which usually protect from infections. Doctors will prescribe a host of medications to minimize the risks, but I have yet to care for a patient who underwent a transplant without spiking a fever, no matter how many antibiotics they were on. As I have said before, it might take two weeks (sometimes longer) until these stem cells start doing their job; during that period, patients are on antibiotics to prevent an infection or to treat a fever that is always assumed to be coming from an infection. Also, doctors will prescribe shots under the patient's skin to push the stem cells to work faster and to minimize the duration of low counts. The quicker patients start making white cells, the shorter their infection predisposition period is.

- **Low blood counts.** Until the stem cells start working and regenerating healthy blood cells, patients most definitely will need blood transfusions (red cells or platelets). I have had patients who refused these for cultural and religious reasons. If patients are against transfusions, they must advise their transplant team to discuss available alternatives.

- **Potential long-term side effects.** These typically won't happen while patients are in the hospital or in recovery mode. It's not possible to include every possibility, but below are the ones we must pay attention to:
  - Infertility
  - Sexual issues (lack of libido, self-confidence, and ability to perform)
  - Early menopause
  - Early cataracts and other visual issues
  - Development of another type of cancer (we call these *secondary malignancies*)

  It's important for patients to know the potential for side effects but to also understand that they do not always develop.

Percentages can be discussed with your doctor if you wish to know them. But one way to look at a side effect with a 10% occurrence rate is to remember that it *does not* occur 90% of the time. In concert with your doctor, you can weigh your options and discuss the potential upsides versus the potential downsides.

I recall performing and supervising an autologous transplant on one of my dear patients whose lymphoma came back less than two years after his remission. His transplant was uneventful, and his stem cells started working within eight days from his day 0. I kept seeing him after that, but five years after his transplant, his red cells and platelets went down while his lymphoma was in remission. We decided to do a bone marrow biopsy, which showed myelodysplasia, a disease where the bone marrow is sick and is not doing its job as a factory, so not enough cells circulate in the blood to do their job. This happened because of the high doses of chemotherapy that the patient had as part of his transplant. Patients who undergo transplants should be monitored indefinitely, in my opinion. While my patient was cured from the lymphoma, we were now faced with a new disease that required treatment.

Complications of Allogeneic Transplant

I tell my trainees that allogeneic transplant is a "different beast": while many oncologists are capable of handling the autotransplants, being prolific and comfortable with allogeneic transplant requires training, a command of managing side effects, knowledge of the nuances of high-risk transplant, and the ability to recognize that patients will get sicker and more complicated. We are bringing new foreign (but ordinary and not diseased) stem cells from a donor to a recipient who likely has a host of issues that led to them needing this kind of transplant.

- **Traditional side effects from the conditioning program**: There is no difference in these side effects from what I have already described, except that we use radiation more often here than with autologous transplants. A radiation oncologist is heavily involved during that part of the program as often patients receive what we call *total body irradiation*, or TBI. Of course, transfusions are also required until the new stem cells start functioning.

- **Graft versus host disease (GVHD)**: This is likely one of the most devastating side effects patients can encounter, although we now have the means to reduce its likelihood and severity. We are introducing new donor cells that might attack the patient's normal cells as these new cells view the patient's cells as foreign or pathologic; this can happen even if the donor is a 100% match with the patient. So, the essence of why allogeneic transplant works (new cells attacking the tumor cells or graft versus tumor effect) can lead to severe and life-threatening complications by attacking the normal cells. If the GVHD occurs within three months from transplantation, we call it acute, but if it occurs after three months, we call it chronic. Why three months? No one knows, but a cutoff was needed to make that distinction, and the powers that be decided that three months was reasonable. In terms of how GVHD manifests and its impact on patients, there is no difference between acute and chronic. Once chronic, though, it can last for a few months or be a lifelong process.

    Transplant doctors usually start patients on medications to prevent GVHD, but the type of regimens used vary by institution. There are some common drugs used across all transplant centers, however. Customarily, doctors check the levels of some of these medications to ensure the right dose for preventing GVHD is given. The FDA has approved some medicines to treat chronic GVHD. Ruxolitinib and ibrutinib are both approved, and doctors will decide if any are indicated in a given situation. Occasionally, doctors prescribe steroids or other medications that weaken the immune system to treat the GVHD. That might sound counterintuitive—why would we ever want to suppress the immune system?—but with GVHD, things are different as the immune system is hyperactive and is attacking the patient's own cells. It is precisely what makes managing GVHD challenging, as we want enough immunity to attack cancer but not too much to hurt the host's healthy cells. While I believe that GVHD can affect pretty much all organs in our body, I think it's fair to say that classically it affects three organs—liver, skin, and colon:

o *Liver*: Patients can develop jaundice; often, the first sign is the eyes turning yellow.

o *Skin*: Patients develop a rash. The extent of the inflammation and its severity varies among patients. My patient I mentioned with the rash had chronic GVHD of the skin, and it was debilitating.

o *Gastrointestinal*: Patients can develop diarrhea of varying severity. Sometimes, doctors are unsure whether the diarrhea is due to an infection, antibiotics, or GVHD. When they are not sure, it is not uncommon to do a colonoscopy and get biopsies that can determine what the cause is.

o *Other organs and systems*: As I said, I have seen unexplained signs and symptoms attributed to GVHD. Patients can develop dry mouth, dry eyes, joint aches and stiffness, lung changes, lung scarring causing chronic shortness of breath, inability to maintain weight, and psychological problems. If a definitive diagnosis is needed, a biopsy of the suspected organ is taken to be examined under the microscope, but that doesn't happen all the time, as experienced transplanters can make such a diagnosis on clinical grounds.

- **Infections**: As expected, the suppressed immune system and the lower white cell counts can lead to higher susceptibility to other ailments, but the types of conditions that can occur in patients who undergo allogeneic transplantation are somewhat different and more challenging than those of autologous transplants. Patients here are more prone to atypical viral or fungal infections, so doctors use prophylactic antibiotics that cover all.

- **Psychological effects**: What patients endure during a transplant would bring down mountains, but I have been constantly amazed at how much perseverance and tenacity they possess. The process and its length and the ups and downs can lead to psychological side effects that must be addressed. These range from general anxiety to depression, stress, and changes in someone's body image and how they interact with others.

  One of my long-term patients who grew to become a friend had a sense of "survivor's remorse" and on occasion would ask me, "Why did I live?" or "Why am I here?" or "I almost died, but I didn't; why?" Oncologists are trained in the art of treating cancer, not in psychology, so a team approach is critical for optimal care, and a patient's mental health should be addressed by other members of the team and by family members and friends. It is precisely why patients must undergo psychological evaluation even before the transplant process starts. There is a multidisciplinary team composed of nurses, pharmacists, social workers, doctors, ethicists, psychologists, and others who meet regularly and discuss patients who are to undergo transplant. This way, the team can surface potential problems and plan early interventions to ensure the best possible outcomes.

Follow-up after BMT

I believe that follow-up after BMT is forever. Of course, this requires various specialties to see the patients based on their needs. Still, recovery from BMT takes a long time. I tell patients that return to employment is not recommended before three months from an autologous transplant and can be up to six months after an allogeneic transplant. Any kind of travel or family function gatherings must be discussed with the medical team to ensure that these are not risky.

At some point during the process, the transplant team will recommend repeating vaccinations that patients thought they'd never need again. Because of high doses of chemotherapy, the immune system is suppressed, and prior vaccinations are likely no longer effective—this can be true even in healthy individuals whose antigens may have waned over time. Timing of revaccinations varies based on the vaccines but is generally within 100 days after the transplant. Your oncologist will discuss these with you, but if not, you should ask about them. Even healthy patients require boosters sometimes.

We know that a transplant works if the patient remains in remission and the cancer is controlled. For an allogeneic transplant, a bone marrow biopsy is done at various intervals to ensure that cells from the donor are present in the patient's body (this is excellent news, of course).

BMT is generally done for hematologic malignancies, but over the past 5 to 10 years, there has been much research and positive studies to show that patients with sickle cell disease, thalassemia, or even some autoimmune diseases might benefit from a transplant. While the indications might differ, the concept of how these transplants are done remains the same.

Oncologists are generally more encouraged when they see a patient with lymphoma (a form of cancer that involves the lymph glands affecting the immune system and sometimes the bone marrow) on their clinic schedule. The reason is simple: we cure more patients with lymphomas than many other cancers, and the experience is satisfactory. The cure, however, is not 100%, and I was reminded of that when I saw my 45-year-old patient relapsing within six months of us celebrating his remission from an aggressive large-cell lymphoma.

"What now?" he asked, and my answer was that we needed to proceed with an autologous transplant to treat his relapsed lymphoma. I told him that I remained hopeful that the transplant would work. Still, I had many concerns about his chances given how rapidly the lymphoma came back, how many disease sites were on his scans, and how bright the nodes looked when his PET scan results came back.

Nothing we did worked; we presented his case at our tumor board, and we collectively decided that the best choice would be a clinical trial. The study explored the efficacy of a novel approach called *CAR-T cellular therapy* (or CARTs) in patients who had failed standard treatments for relapsed lymphoma such as his. I was not optimistic that any treatment would work now that my patient had failed all known active therapies for his disease.

Today he is seven years out from that treatment; he is alive, well, and thriving. By all measures, my patient would not have been alive without the treatment offered in the trial. If someone had described this to me when I started medical school, I would have said, "no way," but here we are with innovation and science, changing lives and curing cancers. So, what are these CARTs?

It's all about the immune system. We already discussed immunotherapy, and if you think broadly, an allogeneic transplant is about giving a patient a new immune system that starts functioning and attacking the cancer cells in the body. CARTs are another form of targeting cancer using immunotherapy.

We have discussed that T cells are the backbone of the immune system for everyone. In certain cancers, these T cells are lazy and are not doing their job. The idea with this technology is that we collect the T cells from the patient and send them to the laboratory, where they are reprogrammed (the medical term is "engineered") to produce proteins (antigens) on their surface called *chimeric antigen receptors* (CARs). They are also expanded and grown so that there are more of them, almost like adding more soldiers to the army and getting it ready to fight. These increased CARs can now recognize antigens on the cancer cell's surface. This recognition leads the CARs to attack the cancer cells and destroy them.

Let's go through the stepwise process of making CARTs:

1. The T cells are collected from the patient. The patient undergoes an outpatient procedure called *leukapheresis*, where two intravenous lines are placed. The blood is collected via one line from one vein, white cells are separated, and the blood is returned to the patient via the other intravenous line.

2. The T cells are then separated and sent to the laboratory. The lab can be at the hospital (some hospitals and cancer centers are making their CARs as part of research) or at one of the manufacturer's sites.

3. In the lab, scientists add a gene for the specific CAR so they become CART cells.

4. The CARTs are multiplied and grown in the laboratory, which might take two weeks.

5. The final product is returned to the hospital, where the patient receives the CARTs.

6. Before the CARTs are given, the patient receives a few days of chemotherapy, which helps lower the number of other immune cells so that the CARTs can work optimally. The chemotherapy is of lower doses so that cancer cells remain in the body, as CARTs work best if there are cancer cells to attack.

7. CARTs are reinfused; they keep multiplying as they attack cancer cells.

8. Careful monitoring is required for expected side effects.

While my patient received CART for his lymphoma, the concept of manufacturing CARTs by engineering the T cells to attack targets specific to the cancer cells has scaled up, and there are CARTs now against myeloma and leukemia. Some are being explored for solid tumors as well.

Side Effects of CARTs

- **Cytokine release syndrome (CRS):** Cytokines are chemicals released in the bloodstream as the CARTs circulate and multiply. This can lead to temporary side effects that can be debilitating and life-threatening. Patients can develop high fevers and shaking chills, become confused and disoriented, and experience a drop in their blood pressure. Often, patients are transferred to the ICU for close monitoring and to get medications to treat the CRS. I recall how little we knew about CRS and how much we needed to educate ICU doctors on the best approach to treat this syndrome. Early identification is critical so that patients are watched closely. To an extent, having some CRS is good as it demonstrates that the infused T cells are working. Notably, the more cancer there is in the body, the more severe the CRS is. Today, experienced centers can easily handle the problem with medications such as steroids. Once we identified that the cytokine IL-6 was the most problematic, utilizing anti–IL-6 antibodies such as Tocilizumab became common. Sometimes these medications are given ahead of time as prophylaxis; doctors decide whether this is indicated on a case-by-case basis.

- **Neurologic side effects**: These differ from the confusion I mentioned above, which is part of CRS. Here, patients can develop seizures, severe headaches, loss of consciousness, and other symptoms that can mimic a stroke or something similarly serious. Why these occur is not clear; they are often treated with steroids.

- **Other side effects**: Infections from low blood counts could develop from chemotherapy before the CARTs are infused, and patients can require transfusions. Fatigue can last for a long time but resolves gradually. There are a host of other non-specific side effects. Still, the most serious ones are CRS and neurologic problems. Much research has focused on developing guidelines and strategies to reduce these so patients can receive this very effective treatment with as few side effects as possible.

Challenges and Future of CARTs

There are other challenges of CARTS, and I am not talking here about side effects. Rather, these include the logistical challenges and the wait time required until manufacturing CARTs is complete.

At one of our tumor boards at the University of Chicago, I recall saying, "I just don't see how this is going to work operationally."

My colleagues countered, "Of course it will; we have been able to deliver complex therapies before. We just need to learn more and figure it out."

I was skeptical; I thought CARTs would never be mainstream because of their complex operations. I am happy to say that I was wrong, and more patients now have access to these life-saving therapies.

How to control the disease until the CARTs are available has become a constant research question that scientists are working on. As you read above, it takes time to manufacture CARTs, and some sick patients may not have enough time since the disease might be aggressive. Also, not all centers are well equipped to handle emerging side effects. When CARTs were made available, manufacturers and insurance companies were very picky about where to allow CARTs to be given. The classic criteria were that centers well qualified to conduct BMT are generally well equipped to deliver CARTs. There were concerns about how older patients might tolerate the side effects, as CRS can be fatal. Still, with more available medications and prophylactic measures, outcomes in older patients appear similar to younger ones on balance.

There can also be manufacturing issues, although these are becoming fewer and fewer. Researchers are now exploring making CARTs from healthy donors, not sick patients. This way, these "off-the-shelf" CARTs can be available immediately when indicated, and there is no wait time. I have seen some promising results with these "allogeneic" CARTs, but none are approved, and they remain investigational.

CARTs are now being moved up the chain in treatment algorithms. Some studies have suggested that they can be better than an autologous stem cell transplant for patients with relapsed aggressive lymphomas. The idea is that transplants can be reserved for patients who fail CARTs.

If you googled anything about CART, you must have come across the name Emily Whitehead, the first child in the world to receive CART for her acute leukemia when she was five. Emily received her care under the supervision of Drs. Carl June and Stephan Grupp at the University of Pennsylvania and the Children's Hospital of Philadelphia who started working together on immunotherapy approaches over 20 years ago.

As reported by Valerie Neff Newitt for *Oncology Times*, Emily was diagnosed with acute lymphoblastic leukemia when she was five years of age. She failed all therapies and was recommended hospice care, but her parents took her to Philadelphia, where she was enrolled in a clinical trial treating patients with a disease similar to hers with CART. She was hospitalized on March 1, 2012, and it took six weeks for her to receive back her CARTs that had been infused in April after she had received various chemotherapies trying to keep her cancer at bay. Emily experienced severe side effects and was between life and death; her doctors almost gave up on her when she was in the ICU fighting for her life as she suffered a severe form of CRS. Blood tests showed that she had unusually high levels of IL-6, and her doctors decided to try tocilizumab, which is known to target IL-6. And it worked. Emily recovered and was discharged.

In 2016, her family started the Emily Whitehead Foundation to help fund more research for pediatric patients (www.emilywhite headfoundation.org). Emily is now 18 years old and thriving. Her photo hangs outside the laboratory of Dr. June to remind him, his staff, his collaborators, and others of the success story that showed how innovations and clinical trials could save lives.

Take-Home Points

- Bone marrow transplantation is now more appropriately named hematopoietic stem cell transplantation, and it involves infusing the stem cells collected from the peripheral blood (rarely now the actual bone marrow) into the patient.

  - If the source of the stem cells is the patient, the procedure is called autologous stem cell transplantation.

  - If the source is not the patient, the procedure is called allogeneic stem cell transplantation.

- There are various sources for allogeneic stem cells.

- Indications for autologous or allogeneic stem cell transplantation vary based on the disease being treated, the goals of therapy, the availability of a matched donor, and other factors.

- Each procedure requires attempting to place the patient in the best remission possible using chemotherapy, followed by a conditioning regimen (high doses of chemotherapy and/or radiation), then reinfusing the collected stem cells into the patient.

- Each procedure has its unique complications.

  - Graft versus host disease (GVHD) is the most serious complication of the allogeneic transplant and can affect any organ, but the liver, skin, and colon are the most affected. There are ways to treat GVHD, and institutions have protocols to attempt preventing GVHD.

○ Some level of GVHD is welcome as this indicates that the graft is working, and it might exert activity against the cancer (a phenomenon called graft versus tumor effect).

○ Other complications for either procedure represent the general side effects of chemotherapy and/or radiation as well as unique toxicities that might be pertinent to some drugs being used.

○ Watching for possible infections is critical as patients are mostly prone to these when they have very low white blood cell counts from the chemotherapy. When counts are low, patients usually require blood product transfusions.

○ Monitoring for long-term toxicities and adverse events is critical.

• CART cellular therapies have transformed how we treat some cancers.

• CARTs basically train the T cells to start attacking the cancer cells.

• Some CARTs are currently approved for certain leukemias and lymphomas. CARTs are being explored in many other diseases.

• CARTs also have a unique set of adverse events and side effects that must be watched and treated if they develop.

CHAPTER 16

Complementary and Alternative Therapy

Common sense is not
so common.

—*Voltaire*

MY NEW PATIENT had a bag full of medicines. There were nine
bottles in there with various names, all over-the-counter (OTC) pills.
All of them had fine print suggesting consulting a doctor if there were
"questions." Some of the bottles contained vitamins, while others
had claims that they boosted the immune system and could fight
fatigue, leading to physical strength.

He was in his seventies and had prostate cancer that had spread
to the bones. He looked reasonably well and was accompanied by his
wife, who appeared more distressed than he was. After we discussed
how the diagnosis was made, I asked him about his medications, including the OTC ones that my assistant was still entering into his electronic medical records.

Patient (with a faint smile): Well, my wife started me on all these tab-
lets two weeks ago when we learned the news. She swears by all
of them, but honestly, doc, I am not sure why I am taking them.

Wife (interjecting): They boost the immune system. Haven't you
heard that cancer happens because our immune system is weak?
Well, I am making it stronger. Plus, you know that your cousin
took some of these, and they helped him.

CN: I understand; I was just trying to know who recommended
these and for what reasons.

Wife: For his immune system; also, there is one that helps with
bone health. I also cut the sugar from his diet. Sugar feeds cancer
cells, so no more sugar. I just made him an appointment for
acupuncture.

CN: We can discuss that in a bit. For now, let's chat about what we
need to do next for his cancer and what tests to order.

My patient and his wife agreed with all my recommended tests
and treatment.

Wife: I must ask you: you're OK with him taking my cocktail of
supplements?

CN: Look, some of these I don't mind at all. There are others that
I simply don't know how they might interact with the treatment
he will be receiving. As we discussed, he will get these hormone
shots but also a few rounds of chemotherapy. I don't know if there
are interactions with chemo or not; could they affect blood counts
or not? I hope they won't, but my preference is to avoid taking
these medications for now as we don't have clarity on whether they
might cause trouble.

My patient and his wife wanted to maximize their chances of controlling his cancer; they never suggested that they wouldn't take the

chemo or hormonal shots I prescribed, but they wanted more treatment, more hope in a bottle.

The National Cancer Institute (NCI) defines complementary therapy as "treatments that are used along with standard treatments but are not considered standard. Standard treatments are based on the results of scientific research and are currently accepted and widely used. Less research has been done for most types of complementary medicine. Complementary medicine includes acupuncture, dietary supplements, massage therapy, hypnosis, and meditation."

Alternative therapy is when patients refuse standard treatment and wish to replace it completely with a nontraditional approach that has not been proven scientifically. The NCI defines alternative medicine as "treatments that are used instead of standard treatments. Standard treatments are based on the results of scientific research and are currently accepted and widely used. Less research has been done for most types of alternative medicine. Alternative medicine may include special diets, megadose vitamins, herbal preparations, special teas, and magnet therapy."

Patients get annoyed when physicians dismiss these approaches; I can understand why. Patients and families might have preconceived notions about certain interventions; there is so much on the internet and TV about these. Also, doctors are viewed as rigid and not able to embrace "different" things. I have learned to listen carefully, to try to understand the rationale, and then offer an opinion. When I was not sure, I would seek help and do my own research to assist patients in reaching an informed decision. In medical school and throughout training, I was not exposed much to these nontraditional interventions except what my patients shared with me and educated me about.

When I go to Costco with my parents (I confess way too often), my mother wanders around by the pharmacy section, enamored by the number of bottles and type of medications. Since she became well versed with browsing the internet and using her smartphone, I get frequent text messages linking to articles on how to reduce risks of cancer, hair loss, aging, and everything in between.

I got curious, so I googled the market size of complementary medicine in the United States and was stunned. It was estimated to be $82.27 billion in 2020 and went up to almost $100 billion in 2021. With a market size that big, manufacturers and proponents of these interventions have little incentive, if any, to do any research that might risk reducing the ballooned market size. Recall, though, that complementary medicine is not just about pills but rather interventions, some of which make complete sense. Others are questionable. The field, however, often combines both under one umbrella labeled as complementary and alternative medicine (CAM). (Patients might refer to it as "Eastern medicine" or "non-Westernized medicine," "holistic," "natural," or other terms.) CAM led to integrative medicine, an approach to medical care that combines conventional medicine with CAM practices that have shown through science to be safe and effective. As the name suggests, some of these practices may not be safe or effective, and it demonstrates exactly what our role as physicians should be: separating signal from noise to help patients understand what they're getting into. Hospitals, universities, and healthcare systems now embrace the integrative approach as it has become clear that patients demand it, and it is best that doctors supervise this as opposed to patients going on their own. This establishes trust but also allows doctors to know what patients are consuming, especially as some of these consumptions might be directly contraindicated with the traditional approach.

So, let's look at what the field and, most importantly, patients consider complementary interventions:

- **Vitamins**: Vitamins are substances that we all need in various amounts and concentrations to keep the body healthy and functional. I can't list all vitamins here, but I have always believed that getting vitamins through natural sources (food or drinks) is best. Having said that, there are situations when patients need supplements, especially while undergoing cancer treatment or receiving specific chemotherapies. As an example, we give vitamin B12 shots and folic acid supplements for patients receiving a chemo drug called pemetrexed (Alimta). I am always supportive of a daily multivitamin, but whatever vitamins patients take, none of them cure, control, or prevent cancer. In fact, there was so much hype on how vitamin D might play a role in controlling cancer, but tens of studies addressing this question were negative. This doesn't mean people shouldn't take vitamin D; in fact, in certain circumstances, it can address other health issues, but it won't cure or prevent cancer. There is so much out there on high doses of certain vitamins that might kill cancer cells—all not true. I have heard of clinics that deliver high doses of vitamin C and others as a remedy for cancer or as an adjunct to cancer treatment. I recommend that patients discuss any of these with their oncologist and be skeptical as to why the oncology scientific community has never recommended or embraced these practices. How these affect cancer treatments and their possible side effects is unclear since these practices are not supported by scientific research. As an example, we know that antioxidants, selenium, and vitamins A, C, and E can help in preventing cell damage, but other evidence suggests that taking high-dose antioxidants during cancer treatment might render the treatment less effective. Generally, vitamins in their normal doses are unlikely to cause harm, but it's important to know that perceived benefits in cancer are unlikely true, and if they exist, are modest at best.

- **Dietary supplements and nutritional practices**: Some supplements are essential parts of standard approaches based on various circumstances. For example, patients take calcium and vitamin D routinely when they have weak bones due to prostate or breast cancer treatments, or to stave off osteoporosis. Patients who have cancers that prevent absorption of certain nutrients from food will require supplements to these. What most people mean, however, by dietary supplements are those taken in addition to standard cancer treatments with the hope that they might aid in speeding disease control, mitigating side effects, or accelerating cure. Evidence that these supplements can do any of these consistently and effectively is lacking. It is important to discuss these supplements with the oncologist as they might interact adversely with the cancer treatment.

Some of the following dietary practices are popularized in the lay press as possibly playing a role in cancer. The list is not inclusive, but is based on the most common questions I encountered with patients:

○ *Red meat*: There is more evidence that processed meat (changed by various methods such as smoking, curing, salting, or adding preservatives) might be linked to bowel cancers when consumed in large amounts over long spans of time. There is some evidence that consuming red meat in large quantities can increase the risk of bowel, stomach, or pancreatic cancers, but a lot more research is needed. It is my opinion that consuming red meat in moderation is OK; I certainly do that in my life, but excessive consumption is worrisome. I advise patients to decrease the days per month when they eat red meat; replace it with chicken, fish, or plant-based meals, when possible; add vegetables; and keep exploring meat-free choices.

○ *High-fiber foods*: Fiber is found in plant-based foods like whole grains, fruits, and vegetables. Whole grains are products made from the entire grain, such as brown rice, whole wheat pasta, whole grain bread, and oats. There is some evidence that consuming high-fiber diets reduces the risk of bowel cancers, and that fiber from whole grains is better than fiber from other foods. It might not always be easy to be consistent with eating high-fiber and whole grain foods, so establishing some patterns and habits always helps. I suggest switching to whole grain or brown alternatives of certain foods when possible. There's no question that adding fruits and vegetables to the diet is a must. Generally, we recommend 30 grams of fiber daily (as an example: whole grain cereals contain 13–24.5 grams of fiber per serving). There are so many fiber supplements out there, but I remain a believer that the best way of supplementing with fiber is through natural foods.

o *Alcohol*: Research has shown some association between some cancers (such as breast cancer) and alcohol consumption, but there was never conclusive evidence as to the exact safe amount for any type of cancer. I usually advise patients to cut alcohol drinking as much as possible and recommend a few tricks, such as not buying and stocking alcohol at home, declaring a month as an alcohol-free one, or using smaller glasses when consuming. The goal is reducing consumption, as research suggests that alcohol is linked to seven types of cancer.

o *Dairy foods and drinks*: My research revealed no consistent evidence linking these to cancers.

o *Sugar*: The number of times I heard from patients or my own family members that sugar feeds cancer cells is more than I could ever count. I don't know where the story of sugar and cancer started, but it is important to clarify. I'll start by saying that no type of sugar, including refined sugar, causes cancer. Because cancer cells grow faster than normal cells, they require more energy. And because glucose metabolism is often altered in cancer cells to meet such increased demand for glucose, it was feared that sugar could feed cancer. In essence, if sugar is needed for cancer cells to grow, then cutting sugar must prevent cancer cells from doing so. This is factually incorrect as all cells (not just cancer cells) require glucose for energy, and there is no scientific evidence that sugar contributes to cancer development or progression. The problem for patients is if they research "sugar and cancer" on the internet, they might come across some sources that refer to sugar as "white death" and state that sugar is cancer's favorite food. A scary thought if they were indeed true; thankfully, they're not. Despite this, there might be reasonable justification to reducing sugar in the diet, because obesity has a link to some cancers (this link is not strong, but it does exist), and eating food products high in sugar can lead to weight gain.

o *Artificial sweeteners*: There is no convicting evidence that artificial sweeteners or sodas increase the risk of any cancer. But a recent evaluation of aspartame by the International Agency for Research on Cancer (IARC, a division of WHO) suggested that it is possibly linked to cancer. Aspartame is an artificial sweetener (brands like Equal and NutraSweet) that has been in use in the United States for decades. Not all medical societies agree with the IARC conclusions, and many have suggested that additional studies are needed.

o *Green tea*: Evidence on the value of green tea and cancer is not very reliable or consistent. There is a belief among people that green tea can boost the immune system, improve health and energy, offer antioxidant effects, and play a role in controlling some cancers. There is a perception that it has no side effects, so consuming it might have higher rewards than harms. It does, however, contain caffeine, so it can cause insomnia; with higher consumptions, it could cause headaches and being jittery and irritable. There have been some studies with green tea on breast, prostate, and gastrointestinal cancers, but these were mostly small and not randomized, and the research did not control for other lifestyle habits. There were some studies supporting the use of green tea in chronic lymphocytic leukemia, but once again, nothing is conclusive. My usual recommendation is that if you like drinking green tea to go ahead but not in excess, and not with the expectation that you're doing so to prevent or treat cancer. You're drinking green tea because you enjoy it.

o *Ketogenic diet*: There is so much misinformation about the "keto" diet that I did a few podcast episodes on the topic, and they were the most viewed and listened to (check out my Healthcare Unfiltered Podcast everywhere). If you frequent any food store, Costco, or supermarket, you'll see many keto options in the food section. A ketogenic diet is a very low-carbohydrate, high-fat diet whereby users significantly reduce their intake of carbs and replace them with fat and protein, leading eventually to what we call *ketosis*, an elevation of ketone levels in the body. As a result, blood sugar levels usually go way down, causing fat to become the body's primary energy source after a few days. The general division is that a ketogenic diet provides 70% of calories as fat, with 20% of calories from protein and 10% of calories from carbohydrates. Researchers have studied the keto diet in animals, with some limited studies in humans, but in my opinion, none of these have been conclusive. More research is needed to ascertain whether the keto diet has any impact on cancer progression, treatment, or prevention. There are some studies on how the keto diet can help patients with diabetes, obesity, or cardiac disease.

The bottom line is that the ketogenic diet is not recommended for cancer care. There is a lot published on various diets, but if you have time, browse through this file from the NCI: https://www.cancer.gov/publications/patient-education/eatinghints.pdf.

○ *Tomatoes and saw palmetto*: I bring this up because my dad was insisting on consuming saw palmetto supplements after he was diagnosed with an enlarged prostate that required surgery. He had retention and was unable to urinate; this was attributable to his enlarged prostate. He shared with me that one of his friends was on saw palmetto and it was "working like magic." I also lectured a few times for Us TOO, a support group for patients with prostate cancer, where many attendees were consuming saw palmetto. The bottom line here is that there is no evidence that any of this helps in cancer care. It's likely that eating tomatoes or adding saw palmetto to your diet won't hurt, but I am unable to find any research to conclusively confirm any benefit in oncology.

○ *Organic food*: I have friends who will not buy or consume anything but organic food. If you ask five people about organic food, you might get 10 opinions. It's impossible to cover all opinions and controversies surrounding this topic, but a 2018 study suggested that organic foods can reduce the risk of developing some cancers. Often, these nutritional studies are done based on questionnaires asking about diet and lifestyle. Therefore, the evidence on organic foods' value is not certain. Organic foods are foods that are grown without artificial chemicals, ideally without exposure to pesticides, but it's not certain that organic foods have zero exposure to pesticides. The bottom line is that there is no conclusive evidence that organic foods impact cancer outcomes positively or negatively. Having said that, consuming food that has no exposure to pesticides is always welcome. As you know, I was involved in the Roundup litigations against Monsanto, the manufacturer of the herbicide Roundup, which I learned was being sprayed everywhere on all crops. With that, its main ingredient, glyphosate, makes it to our food and cereal, and I would propose that research on its impact on health issues beyond cancer is warranted given how commonly it is sprayed.

- **Cannabis**: This is more commonly known as marijuana. I am not getting into the legality of possessing marijuana on the federal or state levels, but I get asked by many about the potential various benefits of using it and whether these vary by how it is consumed (by mouth, inhalation, or spraying under the tongue). Some of the questions are from patients with cancer, while others are from healthy family members. For patients with cancer, I have used medications with cannabis as the main ingredient to optimize nausea and vomiting control as well as to stimulate the appetite. The two drugs approved by the FDA for that are dronabinol and nabilone; I have never used them as an initial approach, but I have used them with other medications. I have also recommended cannabis-based therapies as appetite stimulants for patients with cancer, with varying success. Few of my patients have asked me if it was OK to smoke marijuana to help with their appetite, and I have not objected to that, but I have explained to them that we don't have conclusive evidence as to how effective that would be. I have also used cannabis-based therapies for pain relief, but not as the only treatment—rather, as an adjunct to another therapy. It is important to recognize that using cannabis carries some side effects, the severity of which varies among people. Some experience rapid heart rate, muscle relaxation, dizziness, drowsiness, hallucination, paranoia, trouble sleeping, irritability, and depression, among other possible problems. In healthy people who do not have cancer, the use is at each individual's own risk tolerance, as we don't know for sure the impact of marijuana use on future health problems. This is understandable as studies on this behavior are tough to conduct for obvious reasons. Fear from developing and increasing the risk of lung cancer because of cannabis inhalation, especially in smokers, is justified, but no confirmatory data exist. Contrary to that, a study looked at bladder cancer risk between users and nonusers of cannabis and surprisingly found that risk is actually lower in cannabis users. I tell healthy people that we do not know whether the use of cannabis will increase their risk of developing any cancer.

- **Meditation**: According to the NCI, meditation is defined as a mind-body practice in which people focus their attention on something, such as an object, word, phrase, or breathing, to minimize distracting or stressful thoughts or feelings. I have tried practicing meditation in my life but found it difficult to do, although I firmly believe in its value and do recommend it to my patients and my family members. If successful, patients will be able to relax the body and mind, and this likely leads to better overall health and well-being. The value of meditation has been shown in all fields, including the corporate world, where leaders who practice meditation have been more effective than others. There is no solid research to show how meditation helps cancer control, but it does help improve quality of life of anyone, including patients with cancer, and leads to better coping. In brief, I do recommend it to my patients and their family members. There are meditation apps that anyone can access, including Calm, Headspace, Insight Timer, and others.

- **Yoga**: This is an ancient form of exercise for body and mind. It involves having control over breathing and emotions alongside a stretching routine that focuses on balance, mobility, and flexibility. I was introduced to yoga as a way to alleviate my own chronic lower back pain, and it worked wonders; I firmly believe in its value. I have recommended it for patients with cancer because it makes them feel good and helps to maintain strength, flexibility, and overall better health. I do ask for their yoga practices to be supervised by a professional, as I fear that some postures might hurt them, especially if they're older and have bone disease. Yoga is a natural way to minimize stress and anxiety; it can certainly elevate the mood and enhance well-being. The feedback I received from my patients who practiced yoga was that it helped them cope better with their illness; possibly reduced certain symptoms, especially pain; could help with sleep issues; and, for some, improved their anxiety and depression. It can also help prevent injuries. The benefits versus risk balance favors recommending yoga when feasible with the understanding that it really helps the patient cope more than it helps control the disease.

- **Massage therapy**: How can anyone say no to a relaxing massage? My inclination when asked is to always say yes, that it's OK to have a massage. It's a way to relieve stress and manipulate the muscles so that people can relax. There is no solid scientific evidence that massage helps in treating cancer, but it certainly makes patients feel mentally better. Some studies have shown that it can help alleviate some cancer-related pain. I have recommended it when asked but suggested the light-touch techniques versus deep-tissue.

- **Chiropractic therapy**: I have been asked about this by many patients, so it's important to discuss. The NCI defines this as a type of therapy in which the hands are used to manipulate the spine or other parts of the body. Sometimes, heat and ice, relaxation techniques, exercise, and other approaches are used. I have seen this technique mostly used for back pain, neck pain, joint issues, and headaches. There is no scientific evidence that it can help prevent, cure, or treat cancer, but it can help with overall wellness. I suggest consulting the oncologist before any possible chiropractic visit, as there are situations where patients should not do any of this based on the underlying cancer condition.

- **Acupuncture**: This is a technique where the therapist applies needles, heat, pressure, or other treatments to the skin on areas known as *acupuncture points*, the areas where a needle is inserted to better control symptoms. I think acupuncture is one of the most-studied CAM approaches in research. Most methods use disposable stainless-steel needles into the acupoints, chosen based on the problem or location of the pain. The inserted needles may be twirled, moved up and down at different speeds and depths, heated, or charged with a weak electric current. There are various types of acupuncture (laser, microwave, etc.), but their goal is the same. Since 1997, studies have been conducted to test the efficacy of acupuncture on various aspects in cancer care. One review in 2013, for example, found that acupuncture helps treat nausea and vomiting induced by chemotherapy. In 2016, a small randomized controlled study in 48 patients with breast cancer who were treated with chemotherapy found that acupuncture helped reduce the frequency of nausea and vomiting. Some other small studies showed that acupuncture helped reduce cancer-related pains, and in others it helped reduce anxiety. In breast cancer, some patients might require oral pills that belong to a class called *aromatase inhibitors*. These cause muscle and joint aches, some severe. Several randomized controlled studies showed that acupuncture relieved joint and muscle pains in patients taking these pills, but others have not. A study in 2021 in cancer survivors showed that acupuncture relieved joint pains. In women and men who experience hot flashes from hormonal therapies, acupuncture has been shown in some studies to decrease them. There were studies that looked at whether acupuncture can reduce fatigue-related symptoms, and some were positive. Other studies assessed acupuncture impact on sleep habits, anxiety, depression, and other cancer-related symptoms; mostly, these studies suggested that there is no harm from trying acupuncture, but the magnitude of true benefit can be debated. It's important to note that in 1996 the FDA approved acupuncture needles if needles are sterile, used once only, and used by a licensed practitioner. When I look at the evidence collectively, I have been in favor of acupuncture as long as it is performed by an expert. When my patients ask me, I don't usually object to them trying it, but I do temper their expectations as I remain uncertain how much acupuncture benefits patients with cancer and for how long.

- **Exercise:** I am always in favor of exercise. I have argued that we don't need to conduct studies to show that exercise helps patients, as to me this is intuitive. I do caution patients about the type of exercise and for how long they should or can based on their disease and the treatment they are receiving. In fact, there have been studies that support my inclination; these studies have shown that exercise may help patients with cancer improve their overall quality of life and minimize fatigue and other psychological problems patients might be facing. Exercise also helps mental health, and universally, patients feel better mentally and physically if they exercise regularly.

- **Naturopathic medicine**: I was so intrigued by the concept of naturopathic medicine that I did a Healthcare Unfiltered podcast on the topic with Dr. Nasha Winters (a naturopathic doctor). I wanted to understand that system as I grew to learn that many of my patients were fascinated by the concept. Naturopathy is a program that uses natural remedies with the assumption that these heal the body on its own without any traditional medical interventions. It does embrace massage, acupuncture, dietary supplements, and exercise. What I have seen mostly, however, is that naturopathic medicine is often combined with traditional medicines, with rare exceptions. In speaking with proponents and practitioners of naturopathic medicine, they explain that they treat the whole person—meaning the body, mind, and spirit—and that this leads to better outcomes. I also learned that there are "doctors" of naturopathic medicine who attend a four-year graduate-level school to obtain this degree; their curriculum includes understanding nutrition, CAM, and psychology in depth. Not everyone who practices naturopathic medicine attends an accredited school, and patients often don't verify the credentials of naturopathic practitioners. I also have come across physicians, some of them my peers, who attend courses to understand naturopathic approaches, and they apply that in their daily routine practice when applicable.

- **Music and pet therapy**: When I worked at Advocate Health Care, we had a musician who would visit our chemotherapy infusion suite at least once a week. She would stop by each bay where a patient would be receiving the treatment and ask them what they wanted to hear. Sometimes she would sing, other times she just played her instrument, and occasionally patients would sing along with her. Infrequently, a patient would ask if they could play her instrument, and she always obliged. I enjoyed hearing the tunes but always wondered as to what extent this was helping. There is no doubt that music helps everyone based on their mood. It can be soothing and relaxing and allows for introspection. Likely, it helps quality of life, but we can all agree that it has no impact on cancer directly. A published review in 2021 looked at all the studies using music therapy to help people with cancer; this review included 81 trials with over 5,000 patients. The results showed that music therapy can help minimize anxiety, depression, pain, and fatigue. On occasion, it can generate more hope. There is never a downside to using music therapy.

I recall having a patient in the ICU on a breathing machine and not conscious. My attending physician at the time asked me to keep the TV turned on and asked his family members to play music that they knew their loved one liked. We did; we felt there was no downside. Whether these helped expedite his recovery remains unclear, but I am an advocate of music therapy. Similarly, having pets with patients during their hospital stay can improve their quality of life and bring a more human aspect to their stay.

Patients often complain that their doctors don't embrace any nontraditional approaches to cancer treatment. In fact, this is sometimes why they may not share what alternative medications they are consuming. Explaining that it is always better that we, as doctors, know what patients take is essential. Not only does it establish trust, but the doctor might use this information to ensure patients experience no side effects and to educate about medications that might interfere with certain prescribed treatments.

Some physicians ridicule patients when they use CAM as part of their approach to cancer, and that is inappropriate. Almost all academic centers and healthcare systems have embraced CAM and have built centers for integrative oncology. The key issue here is to ensure that patients do not replace known effective treatments with unproven ones, and for patients to communicate and share with their doctors what they are taking, no matter what it is.

Here is one simple example to illustrate my point. Women with breast cancer who are on tamoxifen might experience hot flashes, which can be bothersome and interfere with their quality of life. Many women were taking Saint-John's-wort, an herbal remedy that supposedly reduces hot flashes. Even men with prostate cancer on hormonal therapy were consuming it. It turns out that Saint-John's-wort affects an enzyme system in the liver called CYP450, which can reduce the blood concentration of tamoxifen, so basically this interaction can counteract the effects of tamoxifen.

Sharing with the healthcare team all the medicines patients are taking is a must. I have relied on my colleagues in pharmacy to tell me about drug-drug interactions, especially when it comes to OTC medications. One time, I was starting a patient on a targeted medicine for kidney cancer, and my pharmacist told me that I should be careful as the patient was taking Prilosec, a known OTC heartburn medicine. There are too many examples to cite, but my point is clear.

I have learned much about CAM and continue to learn. The most important lesson I have learned is to ensure open lines of communication and to not judge patients for taking medications doctors may not always approve of. We must know why they are taking them and understand the data. By working together, patients can achieve the best outcomes.

Take-Home Points

- Complementary and alternative medicine (CAM) are approaches used in addition to traditional anticancer treatment with the hope that these can lead to much better outcomes for patients.

- These approaches can be dietary interventions, music therapy, exercise, yoga, and meditation, among other interventions.

- Please consult with your oncologist before starting any intervention or consuming supplements, as some might interfere adversely with your anticancer treatment. Some supplements, for example, can interfere with the metabolism of the chemotherapy, affecting its blood concentration. Communication with your healthcare team is critical.

Managing Side Effects, Palliative, and Hospice Care

Plato is my friend; Aristotle is my friend;
but my greatest friend is truth.

—*Isaac Newton*

I WAS SEEING A PATIENT with metastatic kidney cancer; he was accompanied by his wife. He was receiving pills that were supposed to treat his disease. We discussed how he was taking the cancer medication and whether he was experiencing any issues. Knowing his bone metastases, I was naturally concerned about bone pain. I had prescribed pain medications during prior visits and needed to check if his pain was improving.

CN: How is your pain?

Patient: I guess OK.

Wife: OK? No, it's not OK. You barely slept yesterday and the night before.

Patient: Please . . .

Wife: Well, if you're not going to tell the doctor, I will.

CN: We do need to discuss your pain. Let's go over what you're taking and what we can adjust.

Patient: I can manage it. I think the treatment is working; it's what you guys told me recently. My pain will eventually go away.

CN: I hope so; in the interim there are things we could do. There are some ways we can help manage the pain.

Patient: I don't want to stop the cancer medicine; I know it's working, and I can tolerate the pain.

CN: No one is talking about stopping the cancer medicine, but we do need to better control the pain.

I could sense my patient's fear of me adjusting anything pertaining to his cancer treatment regimen, as it was working based on the scan we did a couple of weeks before. His pain was not subsiding fast enough, which is not unusual. It is also not uncommon for patients to hide or downplay some of their side effects so that doctors don't halt or reduce the dosage of the treatment they are receiving. There is a preconception that reducing the dose might lead to less ability to control the cancer, and some patients prefer to weather side effects and toxicities so as not to change their program. Cancer by itself (any cancer, that is) and its treatment can cause significant physical, financial, and emotional distress. Addressing these issues is part of the holistic approach to treating the cancer. To optimize our ability to control the cancer, we must pay attention to all these details.

CN: We will work on better controlling your cancer, but also, we need to do a better job controlling your pain. I'd like you to see my colleagues from palliative care who have more tricks up their sleeve when it comes to pain medications.

Patient: Why palliative care? Are you throwing in the towel?

CN: Absolutely not. The team is well equipped in figuring out how we can better control your symptoms; getting their help will help you for sure.

Wife: So, this is like hospice; is that what you're saying?

CN: No, not at all. This is not hospice. Remember when I had to refer him to the orthopedic surgeon to fix his hip because the cancer had gone there? The ortho doctor helped his hip from breaking. The palliative care team will help us manage his pain. We will still treat the cancer with the pill he is on. This is not a hospice referral. Think of my referral to the palliative care team like any referral to other specialties.

It is not uncommon for patients to assume that any mention of "palliative care" suggests that no more therapy for the cancer will be given. I always explained that palliative care is as its name implies: it is a part of the cancer care journey but dedicated to treating the patient's side effects and symptoms while the treatment of the cancer continues. Sometimes, treating the cancer is the palliative care, as treating the underlying cause of the symptoms will palliate and alleviate them. As an example, if the cancer causes pain, then treating the cancer should alleviate the pain. That doesn't always happen, though, and we often find ourselves in need of additional help to optimize symptom control. I have learned over the years that palliative care teams and programs are the best equipped to help patients achieve that.

I think of palliative care as the assistant to the core treatment of the cancer. It is part of the well-rounded approach to treating the cancer, and many research studies have shown that implementing palliative care early on as part of the cancer treatment improves the quality of life of patients, helps ensure compliance to the anticancer therapy, and on occasion might extend life. The palliative care team may also be involved in caring for patients after they complete their cancer treatment as there may be lingering symptoms and signs that can be best controlled with a whole-team approach. But we first must address the elephant in the room: palliative care does not equate to hospice care.

Palliative Care Is Not Hospice Care

Hospice care provides palliative care, but not all palliative care represents hospice care. This is an important distinction that needs elaboration.

There is never an easy way to face one's mortality, but the hospice care philosophy is to accept death as part of the final stage of life. Hospice care is a care designed to treat the symptoms of the disease while accepting that the cancer treatment phase is over. Hospice care is delivered by a team of healthcare professionals from various disciplines, and it addresses all of the patient's needs and symptoms except treating the cancer itself. It favors ensuring the best quality of life under the circumstances and in the final days of life. One might ask, How could patients have good quality of life if we are not treating the disease? Good question.

With hospice, the medical team acknowledges the limitations of what can be done to treat the cancer but also that we can do much more about the symptoms caused by the cancer. We must treat pain, constipation, diarrhea, headaches, and whatever else bothers the patient, but without wasting the patient's time doing X-rays, spending time in hospitals, and seeing various specialists unnecessarily. It's never easy, but often it is the right thing to do when treatment options are exhausted or a patient opts out of cancer treatment.

Hospice care should start when we no longer can cure, control, or treat the cancer and when a patient opts into this phase. On the other hand, palliative care can be provided as part of an ongoing anticancer therapy, even when long-term prospects are good. Guidelines advise physicians to recommend hospice care when life expectancy is less than six months, but I was never a big fan of these guidelines simply because I don't think doctors can accurately predict longevity with such a degree of precision. What I think we can predict is the likelihood of the patient responding to a particular treatment or the lack of thereof. Once we no longer have any viable options, a discussion about hospice care is reasonable regardless of what we might think the survival is.

I cared for a 65-year-old man with metastatic prostate cancer whose best treatment option was chemotherapy, which was projected to improve his survival but not cure his disease. We were having the discussion about next steps; his wife had joined him for that visit.

> *Patient:* Doctor, I have been thinking. I don't want to go through any treatment. I don't wish to receive chemotherapy.

> *CN:* Chemotherapy is going to help you; it will not cure the disease but will hopefully control it for a while. Patients who receive this chemotherapy live longer than those who don't.

> *Patient:* I understand; I know what you're telling me is the truth and I did my own research, but I lived a good life, and I don't want to spend the remaining months getting stuck with needles and coming to hospitals to get X-rays and scans and experiencing the side effects of the medication. I want to enjoy what is left of my life while I can.

His wife wasn't happy—nor was I. Chemotherapy was clearly indicated; it would have given him a few more months of life, and it was the standard of care. I tried to push against his decision; he was young and had an excellent performance status.

> *CN:* I really want you to reconsider; I hate to see you make the wrong decision.

Patient: It's the right decision for me. It may be wrong for others, but it's what I want. Could you please refer me to hospice care, and they can help with what I might need?

Patients always teach us lessons. Giving chemotherapy was the right choice in general for patients with similar disease to his. But it did not align with his views and goals, making it the wrong choice for him. We must always recognize that patients might have different ideas and visions than the ones we assume are correct. Chemotherapy in this scenario may have been the "standard of care" for most patients with similar disease, but proceeding with that choice is not without costs, such as side effects and toxicities that some patients are unwilling to withstand. Every patient is different, and what is acceptable to one patient might not be acceptable to another. As the oncologist, I might have felt that the decision of not undergoing treatment was the wrong choice, but as my patient educated me, it was the correct choice for him, his values, his beliefs, and his wishes.

Considering that my patient had likely more than six months to live, I was hesitant to refer him to hospice care, partly because insurance might not have paid, and partly because I felt deep down that I might have been able to change his mind.

It's important to know that patients can initiate the discussion about hospice, as my patient did. If the patient has decided that they desire no more treatment, it is certainly something to consider. Also, patients can change their mind anytime and request to be discharged from hospice should their clinical condition improve (which is rare) or should a new treatment become available that might benefit them.

Respecting their decisions—even though we might disagree with them—is key to ensuring a trustworthy relationship between the oncologist and patient.

CN: I will make the referral, but I'd like to keep seeing you every so often to ensure that you're doing well and to share with you if any new treatments become available.

Patient: I always look forward to hearing from you—we could talk some football.

My patient lived 11 months and took three vacations before he became too ill to travel in the last eight weeks of his life. I called him on the phone every two weeks; he didn't want to come to the clinic, protesting that he wanted to stay as far away from hospitals as possible—and we talked a lot of football. It is difficult to say whether the chemotherapy would have extended his life or whether the side effects would have allowed him to travel and enjoy the months he did have left.

What Happens in Hospice Care?

My friend's wife entered hospice care when there were no remaining viable options for her metastatic lung cancer. Many patients opt for hospice care in their own home, but I have seen patients who preferred a hospital setting in case they needed something that could not be done at home, or not to overwhelm their family members. There are criteria that insurance companies and Medicare dictate for patients to qualify for inpatient care (because it is more expensive), and doctors would clarify that, but it's understandable that some symptom control in the last stages of life requires a hospital setting.

By stopping treatment when treatment is no longer able to cure or substantially lengthen life, patients might feel better temporarily, and some might even live longer than how long they might have lived had they continued treatment. People might think this is counterintuitive, but it's not. No treatment is without risks and side effects, and forgoing these can improve quality of life, potentially prolonging survival. Hospice care can also help some patients achieve personal goals, such as spending less time at hospitals and doctor's offices and more at home with their loved ones.

There are national standards for hospice care, just like there are for hospitals, doctors, and nurses. Patients and families should choose hospice care that meets high standards; all hospices provide inpatient support when needed, but the goal is to be at home.

Regardless of the setting, there are critical elements to ensure that patients get the best of care under the hospice umbrella:

- Frequent family meetings to update all family members about the patient's current condition. While daily updates are expected, having a formal family meeting every few days ensures that all questions are answered.

- Spiritual care and religious visits for patients who request these services.

- If a patient is at home, every effort is made to avoid ER visits or admissions; coordination of care is usually done by the hospice nurse. Admission to the inpatient hospice unit does occur every so often for various reasons, but one of these is respite care. Family members can get overwhelmed and need help; often, patients can be admitted up to five days so that their caregivers get a breather and are able to do their own self-care.

- Bereavement care. Having counselors who help with a loss, no matter how expected, is essential. The trained professionals can conduct in-person visits, but even phone calls help. These services are usually provided up to a year after the patient's death.

- Medical care is the most essential part. The hospice team is tasked with making the patient feel better when we cannot treat the cancer any longer. I do think that this is the most challenging aspect of hospice care, as some of the medical care that can make patients feel better includes blood transfusions, getting

224 • The Cancer Journey

fluids, and other elements that some might perceive as active treatment. Some hospices allow these if the interventions indeed lead to better symptom control. The reality is that getting blood raises the hemoglobin levels, but it might not make a patient feel better, especially if the patient is not active enough to feel the difference. Patients toward the end stages of life are sedentary and in bed, so the low hemoglobin level is unlikely to be causing any symptoms or distress. The take-home message is that these nuances must be discussed with the doctors as decisions will vary based on the patient's condition. In fact, sometimes hospice care can include physical therapy, art and music therapy, and other interventions that make patients feel better. The goal is to make a patient feel better, not to adjust laboratory values. I rarely recommend checking blood work for my patients in hospice, although I have done so when I felt that we could do something noninvasive that could lead to better symptom control.

A common question I used to get from patients considering hospice was, "What if I get better?" The short answer is that if medically appropriate, patients can be discharged from hospice.

I'll never forget my patient who was in hospice because his lymphoma had taken over his health. A new drug was approved for his disease, and my patient was still in reasonable shape despite being in hospice. I decided to discharge him and start him on the new oral pill that had just been approved for his cancer. My patient lived another year on that therapy with excellent quality of life until the drug stopped working. It's important that oncologists stay in touch with the hospice team when their patients enter hospice care.

My friend called me with a sense of urgency in his voice. His wife was not eating, and he was asking about artificial nutrition (nutrition delivered not by mouth but through veins or through tubes inserted through the skin into the stomach and intestines). He brought this up to the hospice team over the phone, but they explained to him that this was a bad idea. He did not agree.

CN: It's not going to help.

Husband: How so? So, we let her starve?

CN: She is not starving. Trust me, she is not in pain; she is not eating because she has no appetite. The cancer is spreading, so she cannot eat. This is a normal part of the dying process.

Husband: Food will make her stomach feel better; I can't see her like this.

When cancer is advanced, patients' oral intake is reduced significantly, mainly because of no appetite. But there can also be physical barriers to eating, such as tumors in the abdomen or throat, or other barriers. In fact, cognitive decline leads to reduced intake, as patients are unable to eat. It is not uncommon for family members and loved ones to be very distressed watching this, and sometimes family pressure can lead the medical team to administer nutritional intake unnecessarily. Family members fear that their loved one is experiencing hunger pain, facing dehydration, or being neglected, all of which can speed up their death. The feeling of guilt from doing nothing can take a toll on anyone. The most important consideration here is communication and logical explanation to family members.

CN: My friend; I get it; I understand how you feel. Supplements might appear useful on the surface, but they will not make her live longer, and she will not feel better. Giving her something now will cause more problems than benefits.

Husband: Can we give her some fluids, some hydration?

CN: We can, but again, this will not help. It will help you and us feel better because we are doing something, but for her, there will be no difference whatsoever. We would need to place an IV in her arm, and more fluids can cause more secretions in her lungs and make her feel uncomfortable. It can affect her GI tract as well and swell her abdomen. Our goal is to focus on her symptoms, and the lack of hydration in her condition is causing no symptoms at present. You know, I'd be the first to administer fluids had I thought they would help.

There were situations when I did give IV fluids temporarily, but these decisions are always individualized. Patients and their families apply stories of what they have heard from others or from their prior experience to their current situation, but these don't always apply.

In the end, doctors do what they must do every day: *primum non nocere*, or "first, do no harm."

What Happens in Palliative Care?

Getting chemotherapy or any kind of anticancer treatment is not easy; there are side effects that can be challenging to control, and these can get worse if the cancer itself is causing a lot of symptoms. Palliative care doctors are trained in alleviating these symptoms and palliating whatever is impacting patients.

Palliative care is a way to optimize symptom control, and there is no reason to delay starting it after a cancer diagnosis. Several studies have shown that early initiation of palliative care improves overall survival. While hospice care is provided at the last stages of life, palliative care can be offered at any stage of treating the cancer. Palliative care can be given as the patient is receiving chemotherapy, radiation therapy, or any other anticancer treatment, even if the goal of treatment is to cure the cancer itself.

What does palliative care include?

• **Medications to treat symptoms:** Sometimes, these medications are the actual anticancer therapies. In other words, the chemotherapy itself or radiation can be the medications that treat the symptoms and palliate the problem. Indeed, in any incurable condition, the goal is to control the disease and its symptoms, and that is done via chemotherapy or other interventions. These might palliate all symptoms, but sometimes they are not enough, and the palliative care team offers additional insights and interventions to optimize symptom control. However, the interventions that we prescribe might have side effects as well that require optimal control. No matter what the symptoms are and what is causing them, the palliative care team will tackle these in alignment with the primary treating oncology team.

Every chemotherapy regimen, immunotherapy, radiation, or any other anticancer therapy is preceded by medications to alleviate expected side effects. There are guidelines oncologists follow to ensure patients receive all required medicines that reduce nausea, vomiting, and other problems. In fact, these are programmed in the electronic medical record devices so that they are a routine part of the program, but infrequently, these are not enough. That's where the palliative care team can intervene and offer additional options. Tolerance of certain side effects varies among people, and it's important to tailor the intervention to the individual. Oncologists are well versed in managing most side effects, but for the challenging ones it always helps to have an extra set of eyes that might lead to a new intervention. That is what the palliative care team does. As an example, I have used steroids to treat bone pain; these are not a traditional pain medication, but they help in situations like this. Lorazepam (Ativan) and other benzodiazepines can help control nausea, especially before chemotherapy infusions; many would argue that these medications are for anxiety, but indeed they can work to control nausea. The scientific evidence supports integrating palliative care as early as possible as part of the cancer treatment, and patients are encouraged to ask about that.

- **Interventions**: There are scenarios when the palliative care team might recommend an invasive procedure to help control the pain. An example is a celiac plexus block (celiac plexus is a collection of nerves close to the stomach and pancreas), in which doctors inject an anesthetic into these nerves to help reduce the pain caused by pancreatic cancers.

- Many designate the actual treatment for the cancer as palliative if the goal is not to cure the cancer. This is appropriate, but it's not the topic of this chapter where we are addressing how to manage the side effects of the cancer or its treatment. Giving chemotherapy for metastatic lung cancer, for example, is a palliative treatment, and giving radiation for brain tumors is also palliative. Any therapy provided with a noncurative intent is palliative.

It's probably difficult to review every symptom that might require palliation, but I'd like to share general principles to palliate symptoms based on my own experience:

- **Correcting any reversible symptoms**: As an example, there are laboratory abnormalities that will lead to physical symptoms, and simply reversing these can resolve the problem. Severe constipation and confusion occur in patients whose calcium levels increase significantly in the blood. Commonly, calcium is elevated in cancer patients, especially if the cancer is getting worse, so correcting the calcium levels to normal could resolve the constipation and confusion. There are many other similar examples, but the take-home message is to check all laboratory values and ensure that we can correct what is correctable to palliate some of the patient's symptoms.

- **Improve nonreversible causes**: Some causes are not reversible. I think of cancers that have gone to the brain and cause headaches, vision changes, or nausea. We can improve these by giving medications or by treating the cancer in the brain, but if said cancer is at an untreatable stage, there may be limitations to what can be done.

- **Identifying causes of symptoms**: Doctors need to have an open mind as to whether there might be more than one cause of one symptom. For example, fatigue can be caused by the cancer itself, but it also can be caused by the hemoglobin level being down, and the patient might benefit from a simple blood transfusion.

- **Identifying side effects from drug interactions**: OTC medications can impact care, so it's best to report any that are being taken regularly. Drug-drug interactions can cause side effects, and by recognizing that, we can intervene.

- **Differentiating symptoms of cancer from other causes**: The palliative care team will help identify whether the symptoms are from the cancer itself, from the treatment being received, or from a third cause not related to the cancer and its treatment. This is critical as doctors need to know the cause of the problem so they can design a proper intervention.

- **Addressing the psychological aspect**: This is critical for optimal care. Patients can be suffering from depression, anxiety, or anticipatory grief, for example, each causing physical symptoms that range from insomnia to cachexia (body wasting) and other ailments. Sometimes, these are to be expected.

- **Performing periodic assessments**: The palliative care team is now an integral part of the medical team, and periodically assessing whether patient symptoms are improving is critical.

- **Encouraging open communication**: I have found that some patients don't always share how they feel about their symptom control for various reasons, but sharing all information leads to optimal care. Communicating with family members is equally important. Sometimes, the patient's anxiety is due to financial concerns and has nothing to do with anything physical, and the solution is a meeting with a financial counselor. Understanding the patient's values, goals, preferences, and limitations is a principal guide to optimizing and achieving patient goals.

- **Alleviating long-term side effects**: There are some long-term side effects of treatment, which we have discussed. The palliative care team can be involved in alleviating them.

- **Offering alternative methods of palliation**: Much of what we discussed in the complementary treatment chapter can help palliate patients' symptoms. I have recommended exercise to fight fatigue, and the palliative care team can offer music or pet therapy on occasion.

Take-Home Points

- Palliative care is an integral part of oncology care. It is designed to help control the symptoms of patients undergoing treatment for cancer.

- Some chemotherapy and other anticancer interventions are done to palliate the patients' symptoms.

- Discussing the goals of care with each patient is the cornerstone of personalized care. What matters to one patient might not matter to another. Some might opt for less treatment, while others require more therapies.

- Hospice care is instituted when no anticancer treatments are viable or when patients demand it as part of their care.

- Both palliative and hospice care require a team approach.

CHAPTER 18

Monitoring for Recurrence

*If you find it in your heart to care for somebody else,
you will have succeeded.*

—*Maya Angelou*

FEAR IS A NORMAL human emotion. After weeks or months of getting treatment against cancer, there are situations when the doctor stops therapy because the course is completed. Stopping treatment might generate a natural fear that the cancer could come back.

Why Would We Stop Treatment?

- The treatment course designed to cure the cancer is completed, and no additional therapy is needed.

- The course designed to control the cancer is completed. Even when we are not curing the cancer, we could reach a point where the benefit has been maximized, and additional therapy is unlikely to help.

- The course of treatment is no longer working, and there are no other options, so treatment needs to stop and a focus on comfort measures is recommended.

- The patient is experiencing intolerable side effects requiring stoppage of therapy altogether or switching to an alternate program.

Regardless of any of these scenarios, there are times in the cancer journey when treatment is stopped. And as the treatment stops, we all worry about the cancer coming back.

It's impossible not to worry about it; it is part of being human.

My 35-year-old patient had just finished her treatment for Hodgkin lymphoma, a disease that we cure more patients of every year. I have always prepared my patients for the end-of-treatment visit, because there is a sense of anxiety once treatment is done. The anxiety stems from the fear that the cancer might come back, and from the fact that patients will get less medical attention as they will see the doctor less often and will undergo fewer blood tests and X-rays. This change creates more worry that the cancer could go out of control unexpectedly.

Patient: So, now you don't need to see me for another three months?

CN: Isn't this good news? The less you see me, the better you are.

Patient: Not really. Who is going to keep a close eye on the cancer? What if it comes back during these three months?

CN: We are always keeping a close eye on it; you can call and page me anytime if you have any symptoms or if there is anything you want to ask or discuss. But as long as you're feeling well, seeing your doctors and nurses less often is good for you. Who needs to be in a doctor's office?

234 • The Cancer Journey

I was trying to make her feel better that she was starting to get her life back, but there is a real separation anxiety that I witnessed in my patient. She wasn't too thrilled.

Think about it.

When patients are receiving treatment, they are coming to the doctor's office more frequently; their blood is taken and checked regularly; they get imaging studies repeatedly; they are seen by the doctors and nurses more often. There is a sense of security that if something were to happen, the team is right there keeping a close eye on everything cancer.

Suddenly, the treatment is over. No matter how content the patient is and pleased that there will be no more chemotherapy, no more radiation, no more poking, no more of anything, the sense of fear can be overwhelming when the interaction with the medical team is much less frequent than before.

> *Patient:* So, what will we do to check if the treatment is still working and the cancer is not back?
>
> *CN:* Very good question. For now, I will see you in three months to do blood work and an exam. But please call me if you need to see me sooner; I am a phone call away.
>
> *Patient:* No scans? You're not going to do a PET scan, either?
>
> *CN:* Not now. You don't need a PET scan because your last one was completely negative, and nothing lit up. We will do a CT scan in six months.

The decision on how to monitor for possible recurrence is not always the same, and that's important for patients to know. It depends on the patient, the disease, and its potential risk of coming back based on its original stage, how the patient had responded, and whether the patient has any symptoms. Also, how we monitor depends on patient goals and views; these are always front and center in every decision we make.

Regardless of the disease, there are principles of monitoring that we use across all cancers:

- **Periodic visits and examinations**: I have seen these vary among physicians and patients. Sure, there are established guidelines by various medical societies that attempt to frame the frequency of these visits, but I was never a big fan of these, as we need to tailor them based on individual needs. I saw my patient mentioned above one month after her last chemotherapy treatment because I felt this visit was needed to reassure her and alleviate her anxiety. Some patients ask why they need to come in if they are feeling well, and I emphasize that these visits are needed so we can discuss any progress in the disease they once had and to follow up on any side effects from prior therapy. I have often used these visits to achieve the following:
  - Discuss any lingering side effects from the treatment and how best to address them.
  - Review any recent scientific data pertaining to the disease and that might be of interest to the patient and their family.
  - Conduct a focused physical exam as I might discover something that requires further follow-up.
  - Get relevant laboratory data that aids in evaluating the clinical condition.
  - Emphasize to patients the importance of following up with their primary care physicians and other specialists as needed. It is not uncommon that this latter point gets neglected while the patient is undergoing chemotherapy, but it needs to be addressed.
  - Answer any questions that have emerged since the last visit. I recommend that patients keep a log of any symptoms or ques-

tions they may have and share all these with the oncologist so that they are addressed.

○ Discuss the psychological state of the patient and how they are coping with continued monitoring.

○ With longer follow-up, address potential long-term toxicities, such as developing new cancers in certain situations.

• **Periodic laboratory studies**: The type of blood work that is needed varies based on the disease. There are diseases where we follow their tumor markers (blood tests that are abnormal if the cancer is active), but many cancers do not have tumor markers. Examples for tumor markers are checking a PSA periodically for patients with prostate cancer and a carcinoembryonic antigen (CEA) for those with colorectal cancer. Unfortunately, we have no such blood markers for patients with kidney cancer or sarcoma, for example. Also, if the tumor markers are elevated, this might be a false elevation. Elevated tumor markers in a disease with a known marker means additional testing is likely needed but does not mean that the cancer is back. Counseling patients about why some blood tests are being ordered and what will be done with the results is essential. The doctor will order the blood tests that are most relevant. Patients should not be alarmed if these differ from tests ordered for someone else, as both conditions are likely different. Chemotherapy drugs might cause damage to the bone marrow, so checking blood work helps to determine whether this is occurring. So, periodic and individualized blood tests are needed.

• **Imaging studies**: The need for these can vary and may include CT scans, MRIs, regular X-rays, or PET scans. There are no universal imaging recommendations for all diseases. Guidelines exist to help ensure that tests are not ordered randomly, but these guidelines also must be individualized, and "over-testing" or "over-imaging" is not a good idea.

- **Invasive procedures**: Some patients might require these procedures based on their disease. As an example, a colonoscopy is usually done at the one-year mark after removing a colon cancer. Also, there are situations when we must do a bone marrow biopsy to ensure there are no abnormal cells in the marrow. The types of procedures and their frequency are tailored to the patient and the disease. One hat does not fit all.

- **Other less-invasive tests**: You have heard me say this before, and you will hear it again: these also must be individualized. An example is a DEXA scan to check on bone health, especially if patients have received treatments that might have thinned the bones. Periodic visits with the oncologist ensure that the tests needed based on each condition are done.

No matter how much we try, there are times when the cancer comes back. Oncologists know the chances of a cancer returning based on the disease, initial stage, and treatment received, but these percentages mean nothing to an individual patient.

If I told you that the chance of your cancer returning is 20%, I am not certain you'd do anything differently. If the cancer returned, that 20% would mean nothing as it is now 100% in your case. Providing percentages might help if that level of detail aids in deciding what tests to do and why. Otherwise, in my experience, they generate more fear and anxiety. I have always shied away from giving these percentages and focused on what we could do and on the task at hand.

Cancer recurs because these tiny cancer cells that are present in the body somewhere have somehow survived all the treatments we gave. Some way, these cells escaped surgery, radiation, chemotherapy, and/or any other treatment. These cells start multiplying and growing until they eventually form tumors that we can detect by an imaging study, an exam, or both.

There are a few nuggets I'd like to share about recurrence that might help clarify a few things:

- **Local recurrence** is when the cancer comes back near where the original cancer evolved. An example would be breast cancer that returns in the same breast where the lump was originally removed.

- **Regional recurrence** is when the cancer returns in the region of the original tumor. An example would be rectal cancer that returns in the pelvic area and lymph nodes.

- **Distant recurrence** is when the cancer returns in an organ distant from where it was originally diagnosed. An example would be lung cancer that returns in the liver.

How we treat recurrence is beyond the scope of this chapter, as the approach depends on the type of cancer, where it recurred, and the goals of therapy. What is important to know is that recurrence of the cancer does not mean that we cannot treat it. I cannot overemphasize that point because I know that cancer coming back creates an emotional roller coaster and makes patients assume that nothing can be done. In fact, we can cure some recurrences and put patients back into remission.

One of my lung cancer patients had undergone surgery and received chemotherapy for his disease and was being monitored. His blood work was normal, but he was having some vague abdominal pain mainly on the right side.

I recommended a CT scan of the chest, abdomen, and pelvis. He returned to discuss the results. He could sense that I was not pleased with what I had seen.

CN: I see something in the liver. There are two concerning spots on the right lobe of the liver.

Patient: I am very sad to hear the news, doc. What do we do now?

CN: We first need to make a diagnosis.

Patient: What do you mean we need a diagnosis? Isn't that the same lung cancer I had over a year ago?

CN: Maybe, but I can't tell; I only see these two spots in the liver. I suggest we do a PET scan to check if they light up. You'll likely need a biopsy.

Patient: Why a biopsy?

CN: Let's do the PET first, but cancer is never diagnosed on a CT scan or a PET scan. The only way we can verify a correct diagnosis is by doing a biopsy and examining the cells under the microscope.

As you know, the gold standard in any cancer diagnosis is a biopsy. When we see similar abnormalities to the ones that I just described, the odds that these represent recurrence of the original cancer are high, but not 100%.

My patient underwent a PET scan that lit up in these two areas plus a vague area in his colon; there were no other abnormalities. I recommended a biopsy of one of these liver lesions. He returned a week later to discuss the results.

CN: The biopsy showed cancer cells, but these are very different from your original lung cancer.

Patient: What do you mean?

CN: The cells that we saw under the microscope and how they stained look like they are coming from the colon. I think you have colon cancer that has gone to the liver. The PET also showed something lighting up in the colon, which we did not see on the original CT scan somehow.

We ended up doing a colonoscopy, and indeed he had a small mass that confirmed colon cancer, which he was treated for.

This is an important story because the treatment is vastly different for metastatic colon versus lung cancer. My patient ended up having another primary cancer from the colon, and he never had recurrence of his lung cancer. What was interesting is that his colon cancer evolved despite the chemotherapy that I had administered for the lung cancer, making me concerned that the colon cancer cells were somehow resistant to chemotherapy.

Another patient of mine who had breast cancer was in remission. She shared many vague complaints at one of her follow-up visits, and her liver function tests were abnormal.

The PET and CT scans confirmed that there was a disease that had spread and was more likely related to her breast cancer, but once again we needed a biopsy. We checked the HER-2/neu protein on the new biopsy, which was positive, while the original tumor was negative. This information was essential as it provided my patient with another weapon to fight the recurrence, namely Herceptin and other newer treatments targeting that protein. What we have learned over the years is that the molecular characteristics of the cancer recurrence might differ from those of the original tumor, and this observation carries therapeutic implications.

The take-home message is to always biopsy a suspicious recurrence to ensure that we know the diagnosis and that we gather as much information about the new recurrence as possible in order to guide therapy. Imaging helps solidify the suspicion and guide where we might biopsy, but confirming the recurrence is a must whenever we are able. Of course, there are some exceptions to this rule, but these are few and far between.

My last salient point is that not every abnormal finding we discover is cancerous or a recurrence. Prior therapies can lead to scars that we find on CT scans, and no treatment should ever be given unless we are certain of what we are dealing with.

Take-Home Points

- Every cancer might recur. Chances of recurrence depend on the type of cancer, the original stage, the type of treatments that were given, and the patient's overall health condition.

- There are tests that monitor patients for cancer. These tests vary based on the disease and the patient's goals.

- Not every finding on imaging studies done for monitoring is necessarily evidence of a recurrent disease, as patients might develop other cancers or might present with noncancerous findings that mimic cancers on imaging.

- Once patients start seeing their doctors less often, they might develop anxiety due to their fear that fewer visits might put them at higher risk. Addressing this psychological component is critical.

- Some cancers have tumor markers (blood tests that indicate one or more specific cancers) that can be used to follow up on the cancer.

CHAPTER 19

Caring for the Caregiver

From caring comes courage.

—Lao Tzu

I ALWAYS SAW THEM TOGETHER. He never showed up alone, and she was always by his side. No matter what the reason for the visit was, she was with him. He had metastatic cancer and required significant attention as his therapy spanned the spectrum of surgery, radiation, IV therapy, oral chemotherapy, and supportive treatments to get him through a disease that is not curable, but luckily was controllable.

Our visits centered on discussing test results, deciding next steps, addressing any physical or mental complaints he might be experiencing, and scheduling the next visit. On a few occasions, I had to fill out forms for his wife to justify her absence from work or to take an extended time away from her employment if my patient was experiencing more problems than usual or was hospitalized.

One visit, her eyes were red and tired. She looked exhausted, but he was not doing well and needed to be admitted to the hospital.

CN: I am sorry that I need to admit him to the hospital; we just need to do a few tests, give him blood, control his pain better, and make sure his headaches are not related to something serious.

Wife: It's OK; I understand. Actually, I can use some help, so maybe him being in the hospital for a couple of days is not a bad thing.

CN: I know you live far away, so don't feel obligated to be here daily; I promise to call you twice a day and make sure you have all the updates.

Wife: Thank you, I very much appreciate that.

As we were waiting for transport to come take my patient to the admission office, and as I was finishing my notes, I turned to her and asked:

CN: And how are you doing?

Wife: Me?

CN: Yes, you. How are you doing?

Wife: Oh, forget about me. It's all about him; let's try to get him better.

CN: But you need to be well enough so that you can continue to care for him.

Wife: Maybe. I can tell you that I am tired. In fact, I am exhausted. I don't know what else to do; I will take it one day at a time, but aside from anxiety about him, I feel down, and I don't have time to do the simplest things in life so that I can wind down.

CN: I am so very sorry to hear about this. Can I have you talk to someone, or maybe refer you to our social worker or to a support group?

Wife: I'll think about it; I don't think there is anything they can do. I will manage.

Feeling stressed and overwhelmed because someone suddenly becomes a caregiver to another person diagnosed with cancer is an understatement. Being a caregiver for anyone can be stressful, not to mention a person faced with a life-threatening illness that requires so much attention mentally and physically.

I have always cared for my elderly parents. They usually need to see their primary care physician, ophthalmologist, dentist, occasionally the ENT doctor, and sometimes other specialists. Arranging these visits despite my constantly crammed schedule has always been challenging. I developed a sense of increased empathy for caregivers of my patients because I knew up close and personal how challenging this can be. Caregivers can go through a range of emotions that make their daily routine turbulent, and while our attention as physicians is usually directed to the patient who is at the center of our care, directing some of this to the caregiver stands to make the patient's journey easier and smoother.

I could sense the disappointment in my patient's husband when I looked into his eyes as I was explaining her recent diagnosis of lung cancer.

Husband: Could we have done things differently?

CN: I don't think so.

Husband: She had a cough two years ago that lasted a week; I never took her to see someone at that time.

CN: But the cough went away, and she was OK for two years until now. You did the right thing back then, and you're doing the right thing now.

Husband: I should have demanded a chest X-ray or a scan or something.

CN: Please take a deep breath. That is not true. She did not need any imaging back then as she had a mild cough with no symptoms, and then her cough went away. Rest assured that we don't do scans on everyone who coughs. I also know that if she had worse symptoms, you would have taken her to see the doctor back then. Look, she still saw her primary after that episode, and there wasn't anything alarming until two weeks ago, when she had a relentless cough with some blood-tinged sputum.

Guilt is one of the most commonly experienced emotions by caregivers and probably one of the most challenging to overcome. Caregivers feel guilty that they might have missed a symptom or a complaint from their loved one, or they feel guilty because they're not doing enough.

When one of my patients was diagnosed with acute myeloid leukemia, her loving family was always at her bedside when she was an inpatient. I would see her super early in the morning as I made my inpatient rounds earlier in the day, but no matter when I was in her room, they were there. Patients with this type of leukemia can be hospitalized for three to four weeks while undergoing treatment, and I soon recognized that it was not sustainable for her loving family to put their entire life on hold to be at her bedside day and night. I advised them that they need not be there early in the morning and promised daily phone calls and updates. Her older daughter told me that she would feel guilty not being there. I countered, "You need to take care of yourself and your family to keep caring for your mom." The guilt was something I easily recognized in my practice, partly because it is something I have frequently encountered when caring for my elderly parents, as I never feel I am doing enough. As an oncologist, I needed to reassure these caregivers that they were doing everything they could.

Rarely, I would come across patients where I felt the caregivers could have done more. I once cared for a patient who had colon cancer that had gone to distant organs; he usually showed up alone but was sometimes accompanied by his wife. When he got very sick and was admitted to the hospital to relieve his symptoms and to discuss palliative care and hospice, I met his daughter for the first time. She never showed up to any of his appointments, chemotherapy visits, or prior hospitalizations. I later learned that somehow they had become estranged over a family dispute, and unfortunately, she never cared to communicate with him until he was dying. I recall how emotional she was, crying nonstop and never leaving his bedside in his last few days of life. I could tell that she regretted what had happened, and the guilt of why she had never been there for her father was something that would take years to heal.

Before a caregiver starts feeling guilty, they can feel angry and sad. No one wants to get sick, but everyone will. We do our best to stay healthy, but no matter what, there will be a day when our health fails us. When our loved one is diagnosed with cancer, feeling sad about the news and what to come is normal. I would say it's not normal *not* to feel sad and overwhelmed, as long as this sadness doesn't preclude the caregiver from going ahead and doing their usual activities and being involved in the care plan. If that ends up being the case, I categorize this as an expected normal emotional state. I start worrying when the sadness lasts longer than two to three weeks and explore whether professional help or counseling might be needed.

Do caregivers feel angry at their loved ones? Yes, they do. Infrequently, maybe, but they do. I could never forget the semifight that my patient and his wife had in front of me when we were discussing his recent diagnosis of lung cancer.

Wife: How many times have I asked you to stop smoking?

Patient: Many times; could we not discuss this right now?

Wife: How many times did your kids beg you to stop? You promised all of us a million times.

She was getting a bit loud when my patient interjected, "Yes, it's my fault; could we get on with a plan already?"

CN: We really need to focus on next steps and divert our attention to a treatment plan that allows us to get this cancer in check and under control.

Wife, directing her statement to my patient: You failed us all—I am so upset with you right now.

I could understand why she was angry, but that's the last thing a patient needs to deal with. An angry caregiver could exacerbate the personal guilt the patient feels and is counterproductive. Nonetheless, it is common, and it needs to be recognized and addressed. When I see so much anger, I become the doctor investigator trying to determine what's underlying such a strong emotion in the caregiver. Is it fear of losing a loved one? Stress on how to balance everything in life now that everything has changed? Guilt? Or something else? It is important to know the "why," because a successful treatment plan requires a caregiver who is available, sound, and not angry.

It is difficult to encapsulate all the emotions caregivers go through, but one that I frequently encountered was loneliness and eventual burnout. No one truly and fully understands what a caregiver is going through, as everyone's attention is directed to the patient, so caregivers can feel alone no matter how many people they are surrounded with. This sense of loneliness can be exacerbated by how busy a caregiver gets helping the patient, so there is little time to focus on oneself or to even meet friends. All of this can culminate into caregiver burnout.

Caregiver Burnout

We hear the word "burnout" a lot. It is not specific to caregivers, but certainly its impact on caregivers who are caring for sick patients, especially those diagnosed with cancer, can be substantial. If you have not heard that word before, you're probably googling it now, but if you have, you'll know that it is not well defined. I think the easiest way to explain it is that burnout is a sense of self-worthlessness and loss of interest in usual activities. It is mental exhaustion. There are signs of burnout that I was always on the lookout for, but the reality is, these signs are more easily recognized by people closer to the patient and their caregiver. Physicians don't see the patient frequently enough, and not every visit is accompanied by the caregiver, so these warning signs might not be noted. Lack of interest in doing things, especially what someone enjoys, is a sign to pay attention to. Think of a caregiver who has always liked to run on weekends. If that stops happening altogether, it is a warning sign, unless there is a logical explanation. Another important sign is when the caregiver stops caring for himself or herself, which is associated sometimes with trouble concentrating. Some people might lose or gain weight depending on their appetite and how they handle stress. Others might have a disrupted sleep pattern due to anxiety and other stressors. I have seen intolerance to the patients and being short and rude as signs of reaching burnout. The best description for caregiver burnout in my opinion is "compassion fatigue."

Solutions

When facing any problem, I always advise my patients and their families to focus on the things they can change. We can't change that the patient has cancer, nor can we change the level of attention they require. We cannot change that patients need many tests, hospital visits, clinic encounters, and other medical appointments. We also are unlikely to change that the experience will be overwhelming. It overwhelms everyone, so I try to establish realistic goals, achievable metrics, and measurable ideas that can lead to the caregiver being able to cope better with an unfortunate situation.

I asked my patient's husband, "How are you doing?"

Husband: OK . . . I guess.

CN: It's OK to not be feeling OK. How are you coping? Do you have friends? Family? Who helps you when you need help?

Husband: Sometimes; thank you for asking.

CN: Look, there is nothing wrong in asking for help. This is a marathon. Your wife will need you, and I want to help you be there when she needs you more down the road.

Admitting the need for help and intervention is the first step. As an oncologist, I always asked caregivers how they were doing and handling the situation. They're unlikely to volunteer that information and their need for help because they don't want to divert attention from their loved one, the patient, who remains at the center of everything. I always encouraged them to reach out to their relatives and trusted friends when they needed help. Sometimes, it can be that they need help with grocery shopping or other simple tasks. Creating a list of necessary responsibilities and of people who can help is a great initial step, and I have always encouraged my patients' caregivers to do so. Here are a few tricks of the trade that I have learned over the years and tried to share with caregivers when I felt they would be receptive to my advice:

- **Saying yes and saying no**: This simply means learning when to say no to less important tasks, no matter who is asking for them, and how to say yes to the caregiver's self and their needs. The latter is beyond important. Maintain a hobby, go to the gym, go for a run if needed, schedule a time just to go to a movie theater or walk outside or in a mall. Identifying tasks just for the caregiver is essential in combating burnout and keeping the vehicle running. This means scheduling time for self-care. I cannot overemphasize how important that is.

- **Asking the doctor**: There are resources that caregivers don't know much about unless they ask. Home health or even a visiting nurse are options that may be available and that caregivers may qualify for, as insurance companies occasionally pay for these services. Bottom line—if patients and caregivers don't ask, they will never know.

- **Exercise and meditation**: They help, trust me. Practicing mindfulness can help center caregivers on their own well-being, and it has proven effective based on what caregivers have shared with me. It is difficult to quantify how mindfulness and meditation might work for everyone, but it is a well-known approach to relaxation and general stress mitigation. In addition to the mental health benefit, physical health stands to improve. Many mindfulness activities don't require even leaving the house, so the caregiver can be available for emergencies. There are apps, YouTube videos, and other technologies that allow caregivers to practice mindfulness techniques without being afraid of not being available if needed.

- **Counseling**: I'll never forget how resistant my patient's sister was to see a counselor and to get some help when she was caring for my patient, who had Hodgkin lymphoma at a young age. Many caregivers sense that going to see a counselor is admitting defeat and weakness. It's critical to explain that this is not the case. I have always told my patients and their caregivers that when I refer them to a psychologist, it is analogous to referring them to a cardiologist or a gastroenterologist, just a different specialty because we all need all the help we can get. Caregivers are integral members of the medical team, and if they're unable to do their part, the team cannot execute. Explaining this calmly and in detail resonates with most. When my patient's sister sent me an email thanking me for the referral and saying it helped, I knew that we were heading in the right direction. Referring to support groups is equally important.

- **Caregiver's medical care**: My own observations suggest that sometimes caregivers become too consumed with caring for their loved ones that they forget their own medical care, whether it is seeing the general internist or scheduling a screening test. I always gently reminded my patients' significant others when appropriate, "So, when did you see your doctor last?"

- **Taking a deep breath**: None of us, and I mean no one, will ever be prepared for a cancer diagnosis. I have taken care of patients with cancer for years and remain unprepared. So, I tell my patients and their caregivers not to be harsh on themselves. Loved ones will get angry and upset at times. These emotions can be directed toward the caregiver, but never with ill intentions. Patients must not take these tantrums personally.

- **Getting outside**: Study after study shows the benefits of being out in nature. Even taking a short walk can alleviate some of the stress associated with everyday life. Listening to the sounds of nature, taking in some sun and fresh air, and getting some light exercise can improve mood, sleep, and overall wellness.

- **Getting proper sleep**: Quality and quantity of sleep are essential in reducing caregiver burnout. There are aids to use when indicated, but it's important to work toward a consistent good night's sleep.

- **Exercise**: My advice is that caregivers should do what they enjoy. Exercise can be at the gym or fast-walking in a park or a mall.

252 • The Cancer Journey

Being a caregiver is hard. Patients cannot do well and get better without the help and attention of their caregivers. Oncologists must pay attention to these caregivers and ensure that there is no risk for burnout so that the journey continues with the highest chances of success.

Take-Home Points

- Caregivers can suffer from burnout, or compassion fatigue, as caring for someone who is diagnosed with cancer is never easy.

- Oncologists must pay attention to that phenomenon.

- There are a host of ideas and suggestions that can help caregivers mitigate the sense of burnout. Please consider any and all of them, as this is a marathon, and the caregiver's strength and perseverance are needed to ensure the best outcome possible for the patient.

CHAPTER 20

Communication

We have two ears and one mouth
so that we can listen twice as much
as we speak.

—*Epictetus*

THE RESIDENT SOUNDED TERRIFIED when she called me
around 5:00 a.m. on a late February morning. She was the intern cov-
ering the overnight shift in the ICU.

Resident: Dr. Nabhan, your patient Mr. S was admitted overnight.
He is in the ICU and is not doing very well.

CN: What happened? Why did he come in?

Resident: His white blood cells are very low. I understand that
he received chemotherapy in your office 10 days ago. His wife
brought him to the ER because of low blood pressure and high
temperature.

CN: I will be right in to see him. Please make sure the infectious
disease specialist also sees him this morning.

Resident: The wife is very angry. She has been yelling at me and at the nurses. She is saying that we did not do a proper job and it is our fault. She thinks it was your fault that he is that sick and is in the hospital.

CN: My fault? How? What did she say?

Resident: She said that you gave him chemotherapy. They were unaware that chemotherapy can be that dangerous and said they would not have taken it had they known.

CN: Thank you for sharing this with me—I will be in very soon and will address this. Page me if you need me before I arrive.

I had met Mr. S a while back when he was diagnosed with rectal cancer. Cancer of that region is often treated with a combination of chemotherapy and radiation followed by surgical removal of the tumor. Once patients have recovered from surgery, additional chemotherapy cycles are usually administered based on the surgical findings and the stage at the time of diagnosis. Mr. S had very high-risk disease where there was no question that he needed additional chemotherapy after surgery.

I vividly recall our meeting when I discussed the pros and cons of giving chemotherapy. He had an estimated recurrence of 70% within two years, but he also had other medical conditions, such as prior cardiac surgery, extensive prior tobacco use, hypertension, and borderline diabetes requiring oral medications. He had lost weight from the surgery and prior treatment and had become frailer than I had hoped. We discussed the side effects of chemotherapy, and I focused on neuropathy (tingling and numbness in the fingers and toes) as well as lower white blood cell counts, which might predispose him to infections. We discussed the odds of recurrence if he chose to do nothing and not receive chemotherapy. While chemotherapy was medically indicated, that did not mean it was a must for him. I have had patients decline recommended therapies for various reasons. He and his wife were supportive of chemotherapy and signed a written informed consent. He felt strongly that this was the best decision for him, and despite its risks, he was confident of what he wanted. They were both very grateful, pleasant, and eager to get started.

I entered the ICU that morning and walked into his room. He was alert and recognized me but had minimal facial expressions. There were many saline bags surrounding his bed, and as it has always been customary to me, I looked at each bag and read the labels. He was getting many potent antibiotics, among other medications, and was on oxygen delivered by a face mask. His wife was at his bedside, and I recognized his son, who had brought him to my clinic a few times previously.

After reviewing his chart and events, and discussing the case with the nursing staff, I suggested that we go into a consultation room. The intern who called me in the morning was supposed to go home as her shift had ended, but she wanted to stay and listen to the conversation. One of the nurses was also present.

As we sat, I could sense the family's unhappiness and the thick tension in the room. Their loved one was battling a terrible illness and was very sick. I could tell they were more unhappy with me than with the patient's actual ailment. I read the room, and their body language conveyed that I had failed them. I thought they were associating me with their loved one's severe sickness. I summarized the events that had led to the current hospitalization and reminded them that sometimes chemotherapy can have adverse events despite our best efforts.

Wife: We never knew that this could happen. He did very well when he received the chemotherapy and radiation before. How in the world did this occur? You never told us that it can be that bad.

CN: Chemotherapy can bring the white blood cells down, and we all need these to defend against infections. He appears to have a serious pneumonia, and because his lungs are not that great, this is causing more problems than anticipated. He is requiring oxygen and a lot of medications.

Wife: I know that. I know an oxygen mask when I see one, doctor. Why are we here? Why didn't you do something to prevent that from happening?

CN: We did everything we could short of not giving him the treatment, and when we discussed the pros and cons, you all agreed that this is what he wanted. There are limits to what we could do. I even reduced one of the chemo doses so that we can see how well he tolerates therapy before we give him the full dose.

Wife: You never told us that he could end up in the ICU. We would have never agreed to it had we known. I don't even know if he will make it out of here alive; he is very sick.

CN: I know he is. We all are doing what we can to make sure he pulls through this episode. But we did discuss side effects, including infections that occur when the white blood cells are low. We also talked about the risk of his cancer coming back if we chose to give no chemotherapy.

Wife: I don't understand. I cannot believe you did this to him.

She was getting a bit loud and angry. I tried to remind her of the conversations we had, but it was as if I was meeting her for the first time, and as if we never had a conversation before about these possibilities. She left the room mid-conversation, and I was left with her son, who mumbled a few words that I did not understand and then left as well.

I could see puzzled looks on the intern's face and disappointment on the nurse's face. I could tell that the intern was expecting something different; maybe she was prepared to take notes and learn how to best navigate difficult conversations with the family of a very ill patient. I don't believe I served her right, as I was left speechless myself.

Doctors never forget these encounters. By the time I made it back to my office, his wife had left a message with my staff that they were switching their care and were not satisfied with my level of communication.

There is no need to elaborate on the importance of excellent communication between patients, their caregivers, and their healthcare team. This leads to minimal confusion and helps deliver the best clinical care. Good communication leads to establishing trust with the oncologist and the team; this is needed because the road of cancer care is full of surprises, and at times bad days are more frequent than good days. When the patient trusts their team, they will withstand these bad days and cherish the good ones. They will also learn what's under the doctor's control and what's not.

It's also important to recognize that communicating with a patient with cancer is different. The patient is overwhelmed, senses a loss of control, and is facing a life-threatening illness. Understanding that complexity is critical, and the best that an oncologist can do is give time, be patient, listen, and never ever make the patient feel rushed. When I think of the goal of communication, I think of it as a way to establish trust and as a vehicle to convey difficult and hard-to-digest information. Sometimes the best form of communication is listening to the patient and understanding their concerns and feelings. Sometimes, and despite best efforts, patients and their loved ones may not hear all the details. Doctors like to describe this as "selective hearing," but really this is human nature. When we are overwhelmed, our concentration fails us, and we might miss a lot of important details. We may assume that the patient understood, but they may not have. Asking the patient or family to summarize what they have heard is one way to ensure that all the details of the visit were conveyed properly. As physicians, we must ensure that our patients have heard and understood what we have communicated.

My patient left the hospital and transferred to a rehabilitation facility. He never received chemotherapy again and died two months after the hospitalization from a cardiac event. I received a card from his wife after his death with his obituary and a recommendation for me to study more, stop caring for patients with cancer, and think of him every time I dared to prescribe chemotherapy.

I kept that card in a folder where I saved every letter from patients and families who were not satisfied with me. I read that card often.

Almost 20 years later, I can't forget this story, and I still have his wife's card.

I assumed her care after her original oncologist moved to a different state. She was in her mid-fifties, married to a physician, and being treated for advanced incurable metastatic cancer. As she was a new patient to me, I scheduled her for a one-hour visit so that I could get to know her and outline continuity of a treatment plan.

It is never easy to assume care for a patient who was under the care of a different oncologist. As the new doctor, I needed to establish trust quickly so that we could continue the treatment plan without interruptions. I also needed to make sure that reasonable expectations were set so that there were no disappointments in the future. During that initial visit, we had this exchange:

Patient: So, what is the next step?

CN: We will continue the current program. You seem to be doing well on it, tolerating it, and responding to it.

Patient: But when can I stop the treatment?

CN: As long as it is working now, I would continue it. You're taking an oral pill with few side effects. We're fortunate that we have this medication that targets your cancer. I would not recommend stopping it for now.

Patient: So, I take it forever.

CN: Well, until you no longer respond. Your disease is not curable, but it is treatable and controllable, hopefully for a long time, so I hesitate to stop a medication that is working.

I could sense that her demeanor changed. She sat more upright in her chair and became more apprehensive.

Patient: What do you mean it is not curable?

CN: I mean that we are approaching your disease like we would approach high blood pressure or diabetes. We don't cure either, but we thankfully can control them, so we are treating your cancer like a chronic illness, and so far, the treatment has worked. So I would want to continue it. At some point, it might no longer work, and we can change to something else then.

Patient: So, you're telling me that I am going to die from this cancer.

I could sense that I was losing the exam room. I made eye contact with her physician husband, but he was of no help.

Husband: Dr. Nabhan, we are determined to beat this cancer.

CN: I am as determined as you are. I was just trying to explain that at some point, the current treatment will stop working, and we will need to switch to something else.

Patient: I am going to continue the current treatment, but my understanding was that with this treatment, my cancer might go away and might never come back.

I saw no mention of such conversation in the chart. The notes from the former oncologist did not imply unrealistic expectations. I was not sure where the missing link was.

CN: It might go into remission, and I am hopeful it will. I was just explaining that such remission is unlikely to be lifelong, but we have so many tools to fight this disease, and I am optimistic that we can control it for a long time. For now, let's continue for two more cycles and repeat a CT scan, and then determine next steps.

I could sense dissatisfaction, which is a terrible feeling when meeting a new patient. My sixth sense was on point as my practice administrator received a letter from my patient and her husband shortly after this visit, complaining about how I conducted the visit and that I extracted every hope they had about beating the cancer. They recommended I take a course in how to maintain hope for my patients. They of course requested a referral for a second opinion.

I have kept that letter in that folder ever since. I read it every few months. I felt that I failed this patient and continue to replay the events that led to that letter every so often, but I could never figure out what I could have done differently.

The way we communicate is very important. We need to maintain hope while avoiding hype. We must stay honest and deliver hard facts, no matter how difficult they are, but maintain empathy and proper genuine care. Patients want to feel the hope, and our role is to effectively communicate that without misleading them into unrealistic expectations. I believe timing of what to communicate is critical to ensure best results. In hindsight, maybe I discussed the expectations with my patient too soon since it was our first visit and we hadn't established rapport and trust yet. Her oncologist had just left, and maybe she was feeling a sense of loss. Had I waited until we had established more trust, the results might have been different, but I'll never know.

He was 45 and had young children. A disease that normally affects much older people was causing his body and brain to fail. The months preceding his current state were filled with chemotherapy visits, radiation, tests, and more bad news than good. His wife and two young children didn't appear to grasp the gravity of the situation. How could they? His 80-year-old dad whom I met during a few visits mumbled one time to me, "No father should ever bury his son."

It's customary to ask for a family meeting to explain where things are and share expectations with the patient and the family. I proposed a meeting with a plan to discuss palliative care and a hospice referral. We planned on 5:00 p.m. in the hospital room where he had been admitted three days prior to control a relentless cancer pain. His wife and dad were at his bedside as he laid down, appearing worn out, pale, thin, and exhausted. His mother was watching his children and wasn't in attendance.

I have learned over the years that the best approach to starting these difficult end-of-life conversations is to get an understanding on whether the patient and family know the current state.

I opened the meeting.

CN: Truly appreciate meeting now. I know the past few months have been anything but easy. I haven't shared any good news as of late because we haven't had any. But maybe help me understand how you think the situation is. What's your understanding of where we are now?

Wife: The last treatment did not work; I get that. He is having lots of pain because the last chemo did not work. You must give him blood because he is anemic, and this is causing his fatigue and weakness. His pain medications are making him sleepy, but maybe we can adjust them. We are hoping that the new treatment might work better and help him keep fighting.

CN: Thank you for that. How about you? What's your understanding of what's going on?

Patient (while sleepy): I agree. I am ready for the next round. Hit me up and let's kick this cancer away.

CN: I don't believe we have choices that will give you any meaningful results. The remaining options can cause more problems and side effects with very little benefit, if any. I can't just prescribe anything. I recommend that we focus on your symptoms and have you experience no pain.

Wife: Yes, we don't want him in pain, but are you giving up on him? On us? On his children?

CN: Absolutely not. I am just suggesting that the treatments that we have won't work, so we need to change course and set realistic expectations. We need to shift from controlling the cancer to controlling the symptoms the cancer is causing, but we need to intentionally ignore that the cancer exists. So, we don't treat the cancer, only its symptoms. It's not because we don't want to treat the cancer; it's because I don't think we have anything that would work.

The patient was getting sleepy; I wasn't sure how much information he was absorbing.

Wife: So, you are giving up?

CN: I am just trying to set reasonable goals, trying to make sure that we all have the same objectives. We could choose some chemo agent and give it, but the chances of it helping are nearly zero percent, and the chances of it causing problems and side effects are nearly 100 percent. I don't think there is much that we can do at this point to alter the course of the disease.

Conversations about end-of-life care are challenging and can be heartbreaking. Every family is different, with variable dynamics and principles. Making decisions to stop therapy is never easy and requires a better understanding of the patient's goals. Doctors must know these goals before the patient is too sick to make critical decisions and is unable to verbalize their goals. Waiting until someone is too ill will lead to inaccurate choices as different circumstances dictate decisions. What is most difficult is to maintain hope in dire situations. I have learned that the best way to do so is to ensure that communication channels are open and to shift the focus of the treatment based on new findings or inputs.

How do we maintain hope? In my experience, we do so by identifying new goals and setting our hopes high that we can achieve these new goals. I told my patient and his family that my goal was for him to spend most of his time outside the hospital with his loved ones as alert as possible and pain-free. These were our goals. We shifted our hope from defeating the cancer to achieving new goals. As we continued the conversation, we agreed on realistic goals. Getting the family and the patient there is what leads to a successful hope in dire situations.

There are ways to maintain hope even in the worst situations, but only by shifting goals realistically and communicating that effectively.

One day, I walked into the exam room to find more people than chairs. My medical assistant had warned me that there were a "lot of people" with Mr. V, who was seeing me as an initial visit for his newly diagnosed metastatic cancer. It was a disease that I had some treatments in my toolbox for. Mr. V was an immigrant who had moved to Chicago 30 years earlier. He worked hard and had built a wonderful family, including two caring daughters who lived nearby. They both accompanied him to this first visit along with two sons-in-law. His wife spoke very little English but had a nice smile on her 75-year-old face; she sat on a chair while Mr. V was sitting on the exam table. The sons-in-law were standing, and their wives (my patient's daughters) sat on the remaining two chairs in my now-crowded exam room.

I started by asking questions, which were most often answered by one of the daughters. Mr. V's English was not perfect, but he could answer some questions. For others, he would look at one of his daughters, seeking help in answering. For the most part, he was nodding as his elder daughter took charge. She was the person in the room doing most of the talking.

I reached a decision on the best next step and started discussing the treatment plan. Subconsciously, I was a bit concerned as to whether all my statements were being translated correctly to him. I had no evidence to the contrary, except my intuition. The daughter was asking more questions about efficacy of the proposed treatment and side effects. At some point during the conversation, I had the feeling that she would make the final decision for him, and that concerned me. I needed to make sure that my patient was knowledgeable of what he would be on and the pros and cons of such therapy, but I did not feel I was connecting with him. It was almost a two-way conversation between me and his daughter, who sensed that I was becoming a bit uncomfortable with that exchange.

Daughter: It is OK; I will make these decisions.

CN: But even if you had the power of attorney, he needs to decide unless he explicitly says that you are the decision-maker.

Daughter: I understand, but he wants me to make all treatment decisions, even now. He trusts me.

CN: May I ask him? I need to hear that from him.

I shifted my chair toward him and asked gently if this was the case. While his English wasn't perfect, he understood what I was asking. In broken English, he said, "Yes, doctor—my daughter decides. She knows better what I want, and she is smarter than me."

CN: Even when it comes to deciding on chemotherapy?

Patient: Yes.

This might be surprising in Western cultures, but it is not that unusual in different parts of the world. I make many decisions for my parents, who want me to decide on all aspects of their medical care. Sometimes, my mother tells me, "I don't want to know."

Doctors must accept different cultures and accommodate beliefs that are not aligned with their own. Language barriers and beliefs can impair communication, and oncologists need to adjust to ensure that best communication is maintained despite these challenges. This is mostly critical when beliefs are not aligned with best medical judgment.

I have had patients who designated a family member or a trusted friend to make decisions. I also had patients who wanted to know every detail. But most patients fall in the middle.

I can't ever forget the day I met my young patient who was diagnosed with an aggressive form of leukemia, a blood cancer that is often fatal. As a young man who had never been sick, the sense of losing control over his life trajectory was evident and exhibited by his reluctance to follow much of the proposed medical advice.

When I met his dad for the first time, he made it clear that he wasn't a big fan of mine, suggesting that he wanted second, third, and fourth opinions.

CN: It is important that you get all the opinions you need. I can help arrange these, but time is of the essence, and we do need to start treatment rather urgently.

Father: I get it. Please connect me with other experts in this disease.

CN: He is too sick to leave the hospital, but we can arrange for a hospital-to-hospital transfer, or he can see one of the other oncologists who practices here.

Father: OK; I can see someone who is here.

I took care of arranging the second opinion, which concurred with my recommendations. It became clear to me that ensuring that the patient and his family were in full control of the decision-making process was critical moving forward. While this is always important, my sense was that it was more important here than other encounters I'd had.

We often speak about shared decision-making. The principle is simple. When it comes to decisions regarding medical care, patients must remain in the center and be involved in deciding what to do every step of the way.

This is an excellent and important idea, but it also assumes that patients and physicians can process the information equally and that patients can easily understand the nuances of complex decision-making, something that takes years of training to reach such a level of expertise.

I started seeing my leukemia patient twice a day, a change from my routine of once daily before clinic. When someone was sicker than usual, I would see them more frequently, as there are many moving parts to medical decisions that need to happen daily and sometimes hourly. I met with his family daily, and when his dad was not present, I would call him and discuss the details.

I knew that no matter what, my patient and his family would struggle to understand every single detail of the treatment decisions, but I wanted to give them the sense of control over every decision. This strengthens trust through frequent communication and dialogue. Within a couple of weeks, I could sense a change in the tone of our conversations whereby trust had been established.

Some patients and families want frequent communication, while others might choose it to be less frequent. But everyone needs to sense the feeling of control. The feeling of losing control over decision-making can be detrimental. Losing control during the most vulnerable time of someone's life is traumatic, and patients need to be open about what would make them feel more comfortable and at ease.

To this day, I stay in touch with my patient, who successfully navigated a complicated leukemia treatment and for all practical purposes has been cured. He often teases me about how his dad become a big fan.

Physicians talk about shared decision-making all the time. As I said above, the concept or principle is obvious. Medical decisions should be joint ones between patients and their medical team, but this concept can be elusive as patients might not be aware of or able to understand the nuances of some of these decisions.

When I was a fellow rotating through the lymphoma clinic, I would try to learn every aspect of oncology care, including how best to communicate with patients.

We were seeing a patient with non-Hodgkin lymphoma. The type of lymphoma this patient had was indolent, meaning it was slow growing but likely not curable. There were many options to treat this kind of lymphoma, and I was listening to my attending who told the patient, "There is a buffet of choices." She went on to discuss various treatment options and explained the side effects of each and what to expect.

Patient: Doctor, what would you take if you were me?

This is a very common question that patients ask, but it is impossible to answer. What matters to one patient might not matter to others. At the same time, it is extremely challenging to put patients in a situation where they must select therapy without ever having undergone the training required to decide on optimal therapy.

In my view, shared decision-making is about the patient agreeing with or refuting the medical recommendation, not about deciding on the medical recommendation itself.

I can't ever forget my wonderful 75-year-old patient who required chemotherapy to extend her life and control her cancer.

Patient: Will I lose my hair?

CN: Unfortunately, you likely will lose your hair.

Patient: I don't want it, then. I won't ever want to be bald. I won't take it; give me something else.

CN: But this is the one that can help you the most, and it will likely make you live longer than any other treatment. There are studies—

Patient: Sorry to interrupt you; I don't doubt that this is the best for many patients, but it is not for me. I would rather die a year earlier with my hair intact than live longer with no hair.

Her daughter, who was in the room, looked very disappointed. I prescribed a different chemotherapy that ensured my patient wouldn't suffer from hair loss.

I made the decision that she needed chemotherapy, but the shared decision-making led us to decide which type of chemotherapy regimen she was most comfortable with.

How to Communicate?

- Patients must speak up. Ask every question you have; ask and ask often, and if you're not getting answers, ask again. Ask the same question different ways if you need to. Your doctor and the medical team are there to make the journey easier, and they must fulfill their end of the bargain.

- Communication is a continuum. A doctor needs to advise you on medical decisions when it comes to selecting a cancer therapy but also guide you with other life events while you're dealing with cancer. You may not like what they are saying, but it is their duty to tell you the truth and to help you make good medical choices that take your values into consideration. Say you need to go to a wedding, or had planned a lifetime vacation. You and your doctor need to work as a cohesive team to ensure you get to do what you wish. Your doctor needs to accommodate changes in your life or needs. What matters might change as we progress in the cancer journey, and patients need to communicate changes in their preferences so that the medical team can adjust accordingly.

- Doctors must be transparent about available options or the lack thereof. Discussing absence of treatment choices is always difficult, whether someone is 15, 50, 60, or 80 years old. We all want to live and to live well, but there comes a time when we have no other choices, and the toolbox empties out. Patients rely on their doctors to communicate effectively about this and about what must be done next. Communicating when "goals of care" change is something that we need to teach our trainees more of. I don't recall having classes or being taught how best to break good or bad news. I developed these skills from witnessing my teachers and attendings while seeing patients with them and added my own flavor as I gained more experience with time.

- Communicating with caregivers is essential. Caregivers are partners in this journey, and they are the eyes and ears of the doctor as to what happens at home. A caregiver is often a notetaker, question-asker, and medication administrator. They should be part of the discussion whenever possible.

- There can be cultural differences and language barriers with your doctor. Every hospital has someone who can translate information to patients' mother tongues, so patients can ask for a translator if they don't have someone accompanying them who speaks English.

- There are times when patients might not fully understand the plan; this is OK. They must ask, and after processing the information, they should ask again. Patients must end up on the same level as the doctor to ensure that they know what is happening every step of the way. Problems arise when patients don't fully comprehend the goals of treatment. Are we trying to cure this cancer? Control it? What are the chances of either goal?

- Patient-friendly brochures to explain detailed information are widely available. There are usually brochures written in various languages, but if not, there are ways to obtain these through community services and patient support groups.

- Patients must not be afraid of taking too much of the doctor's time. Doctors are here to answer inquiries and hopefully to spend as much time as needed doing so. There were times when my patients brought a list of 40 questions with them to a follow-up visit, and I did have to ask them to prioritize and choose the top 10 because we wouldn't have time to get through all of them during that particular visit. But I promised that I would call after my clinic ended to go over the remaining ones that we didn't get to address. This always went well. Patients know that we might not be able to address everything in one visit, and often there are more pressing questions that require immediate attention.

Optimizing Communication

There are doctors who get very upset when patients are referred to as "customers," and I can understand why. There is a sense that this might downgrade the level of the noble relationship between doctors and patients. I never viewed it this way. Ultimately, patients consume healthcare products, whether these are medications, tests, or simple doctor's visits. I often think that adding the label of "customer" or "consumer" might lead healthcare professionals to care more about

simple but important things like wait times, callbacks, and other logistical challenges that patients usually complain about.

As I think of how best to improve the level of communication between patients and their healthcare team, I propose this itemized list:

- Patients should write down a list of the questions they plan on
  asking at every visit. As patients, we all know the questions that
  are most pressing and need to be addressed quickly. These should
  be prioritized.

- It's best for patients to have someone else with them at visits. "I
  want an extra set of ears," I would say. Sometimes, patients don't
  hear everything—not because they're not listening but because
  they're overwhelmed. Having someone they trust with them is
  vital. This is not needed at every visit but important in the crucial ones, such as the first chemotherapy infusion visit, the first
  oncology visit, or when the doctor is planning to discuss findings
  of imaging studies to check whether the cancer is responding to
  treatment.

- Patients should write down appointments, dates of tests, and results in a journal that they can refer to when needed or share
  when getting second opinions.

- It is OK to ask the doctor if the visit can be recorded. As I have
  mentioned, my patients recorded me numerous times, and I always embraced it. I once had a patient whose daughter would
  film the entire visit on her mobile phone, including my exam,
  and she would send that to her brother who lived far away. I never
  minded that. But I always wanted to be asked first. I did have to
  call my hospital legal office to ensure that this was allowed, and
  they told me that it was my choice, so I agreed. If the doctor re-
  fuses, it might be due to a hospital policy. All doctors must adhere to the policies and procedures of the healthcare systems
  they belong to.

- Patients must be their own advocates. If they don't understand something, they should ask questions until they understand.

- I always asked my patients to repeat to me what they understood and heard. If a doctor does not ask for this, patients can say, "Can I tell you what I think I heard?" or something of that nature.

The journey of cancer care is never easy, but clear and effective communication will make it easier, less bumpy, and more predictable.

Take-Home Points

- Optimizing communication between patients and their healthcare team is essential for achieving best results, minimizing disappointments between both sides, and setting realistic expectations.

- In communicating, doctors can maintain hope while avoiding hype.

- Respecting and understanding different cultures is critical for best communication.

- Even if patients don't speak English, practices and hospitals have translators to help communicate the plan and next steps. Ask for one if needed.

- If possible, have someone with you during essential oncology visits so they can provide an extra set of ears and remind you about what you may have missed, as seeing the oncologist can be overwhelming.

CHAPTER 21

Survivorship and the Emotional Journey of Cancer

Change is the law of life. And those who look only
to the past or present are certain to miss the future.

—*John F. Kennedy*

MY 50-YEAR-OLD PATIENT was always pleasant, no matter what
the issues were. He had an optimistic view on life despite being diagnosed with metastatic lung cancer. He was divorced, had one son, and
was employed when we met. I prescribed chemotherapy, which he
responded very well to; this was followed by one of the oral targeted
treatments, as we found that his cancer had a mutation that predicted
he would benefit.

He had been on that pill for about a year when he saw me for a routine visit. We would normally do blood work, I would check for any
side effects, and we would do a scan if needed. As we were finishing,
we had this exchange:

Patient: Dr. Nabhan, what do I do with my 401(k)?

CN: Pardon me?

Patient: What am I supposed to do with my 401(k)? I have some money I have been putting there. But why should I contribute?

CN: So you can save for retirement?

Patient: Come on—what retirement? I have lung cancer that has spread, so why not enjoy the money? There's no way I will be around when I can collect that money.

I was completely unprepared for that question; I had not been asked it before. I thought quickly and could see what my patient was saying. Knowing him and his personality, I could also understand why he was asking.

CN: I really don't know what to tell you; that's an individual decision, and probably one you would make with a financial advisor and your family.

Patient: What would you do if you were me? Would you still put aside a chunk of money each month in an account that you may never have access to in your lifetime?

CN: It's probably something that your son can benefit from in the future.

Patient: I will contribute much less; I need to live whatever months or years I have left for me.

I still remember how deeply I thought about my patient's question that night. Almost 15 years later, this visit remains fresh in my memory. It highlights that there are so many aspects to patients' lives beyond treating the cancer itself. Life must go on despite the diagnosis; it's what I call *survivorship*.

Researchers have argued about the definition of survivorship and when and how this is labeled. My simple mind proposes that the term "cancer survivorship" starts from the time of diagnosis as opposed to the time of completing therapy. There are so many elements of living that patients must deal with the minute a diagnosis is rendered, and healthcare professionals must recognize that patient needs must be attended to in a timely and appropriate manner.

Indeed, on their website the NCI defines survivorship as follows:

> In cancer, survivorship focuses on the health and well-being of a person with cancer from the time of diagnosis until the end of life. This includes the physical, mental, emotional, social, and financial effects of cancer that begin at diagnosis and continue through treatment and beyond. The survivorship experience also includes issues related to follow-up care (including regular health and wellness checkups), late effects of treatment, cancer recurrence, second cancers, and quality of life. Family members, friends, and caregivers are also considered part of the survivorship experience.

A cancer survivor is anyone dealing with cancer as a patient. This can be someone who has just started treatment, has just received a diagnosis, is undergoing long-term chronic therapy, or has completed all treatments and is on observation and monitoring. Some patients don't like these definitions and view them as labels, but the terms have been accepted by oncology societies and governmental bodies as this helps generate funds to study long-term impacts of cancers on life and what can be done to mitigate side effects beyond those generated from the treatment itself. Doctors should be attuned to their patients and address these issues based on individual needs and beliefs.

What's important is to recognize the problems and their magnitude. To put things in perspective, recent figures suggest that while almost 2 million people in the United States are diagnosed with cancers annually, there are about 18 million people with a history of cancer who live in the United States, which is a sharp increase from 3 million people living with the disease back in 1971. About two-thirds of cancer survivors have lived five or more years after diagnosis, and in fact, 18%–20% have survived two decades or more since initial diagnosis. While most cancer deaths occur in patients over the age of 65, 64% of cancer survivors are age 65 or older. Of course, these statistics vary based on the disease and the patient, and these numbers may mean nothing to an individual person because it's impossible to think in these terms when faced with a critical illness. Why patients are doing better is multifactorial: early detection because of screening; better treatment options; improved therapeutic choices; enhanced technology, whether for surgery, radiation, or targeted approaches; better supportive care and the ability to control and treat side effects; and innovative clinical trials, among other factors.

What Patients Might Deal With

Every person is different, so I will summarize my observations from practicing oncology for almost two decades and caring for many patients facing cancer.

Psychological Issues

"Why am I still here?" he asked me after undergoing grueling autologous transplantation for his relapsed large-cell lymphoma.

> CN: You're here because you're meant to be here; let's think about what you want to accomplish moving forward.

> Patient: I may not have many years.

CN: Let's be optimistic: your transplant has been successful; there's no reason to assume the worst. Soon your hair will grow back, and you can return to work.

Patient: I am not so sure.

CN: I am. I also think you'd benefit from speaking to your psychologist; I recall she helped you a lot when we were preparing for the transplant.

One of my long-standing patients whom I developed a close relationship with was on the verge of dying before an allogeneic transplant saved his life. He would touch base with me every so often, and on occasions, we would meet and have coffee. His care was transitioned to a transplant expert, but we maintained this relationship for years after his transplant. He started his own company and was doing well financially; however, he had challenges in maintaining close relationships, and although he dated, he was unable to maintain a long-term girlfriend.

We were having coffee one time, and he looked at me asking the same question, "Why am I here?"

CN: Pardon me?

Patient: I don't know why I am here. Why did others die and I did not?

I have seen this "survivor's guilt" many times. It is a true phenomenon and can be challenging to address. Emotions are heavy, and some patients struggle in expressing them while doctors are challenged in how to address them. This phenomenon is magnified as patients learn about others who didn't make it and succumbed to the disease; making sense of all this is no easy feat. Many cancer survivors experience this guilt, and I find it imperative to bring it out in the open versus hiding it or being ashamed of it.

Survivorship is an unpredictable emotional roller coaster. Patients move from being seen by doctors and nurses all the time to having distant visits and infrequent blood draws and tests. This can lead to significant anxiety and fear, as we have discussed. I have found that psychological counseling is essential in these scenarios and have always offered it to my patients. I work with my patients to transform the guilt into gratitude. This is not to say that patients are not grateful, but extra work is needed to make sure these emotions are transferred into positive ones. Time is usually needed for patients to start recognizing the silver lining, and as time passes, the guilt hopefully subsides.

Anxiety about cancer recurrence is to be expected. Not experiencing anxiety is impossible, but the goal is to make sure worries don't interfere with usual activities and daily living. If anxiety starts interfering with daily living, referral to psychologists and/or psychiatrists is needed. There are various reasons why patients can become very anxious, but physical symptoms that might imply potential recurrence are among the most common. Being anxious about the possibility that side effects from treatment may not resolve is also common.

Depression is another mental illness that cancer survivors might suffer from. Patients can feel sad, experience distress, lack interest in daily activities, and become withdrawn or angry. These feelings might imply an underlying depressive disorder that needs to be addressed. I think the occasional feeling of hopelessness in someone who is undergoing grueling cancer treatments is normal, but when this interferes with life, especially after completing treatment, it can be a sign of clinical depression that requires medical attention.

Currently, the American Society of Clinical Oncology (ASCO) recommends screening patients for anxiety and depression starting at the time of diagnosis. Screening is also recommended during and after treatment; it is usually in the form of a questionnaire that patients respond to when they're in the office. The idea is that screening can catch problems early and allow professionals to intervene with either medical or behavioral interventions.

The most severe form of these psychological issues is suicidal ideation and sometimes suicide. I lost a patient who had terminal small-cell lung cancer to suicide. He was undergoing chemotherapy when he was found dead in his garage with a self-inflicted gunshot wound. Since then, I have paid much more attention to psychological issues. It is true that he had an incurable illness with limited survival, but none of us expects our patients to take their own lives. I viewed that incident as a failure on my part and have always counseled my patients on anxiety and depression.

Physical Issues

Survivors of cancer deal with side effects of the treatment as well as physical symptoms that the cancer might be causing. Some of these side effects are acute, meaning they occur at the time of diagnosis or during treatment, but others are chronic and linger for a long time after completing therapy.

Also, there is the potential for future physical side effects and other illnesses. Some scenarios develop as more time lapses, since certain adverse events don't manifest for months and sometimes years after completing treatment.

We already discussed navigating short-term side effects and adverse events as these vary based on the treatment and the disease itself. For long-term issues, ASCO has issued various long-term follow-up care plans that vary based on the disease state. In other words, patients who have completed breast cancer treatment, for example, might have a different follow-up care plan than patients who have completed treatment for diffuse large B-cell lymphoma. Variations depend on the stage of disease, goals of care, comorbidities, and the treatments patients received. General themes for these treatment plans include:

- Follow-up with routine examinations and blood work to detect recurrence of the cancer as early as possible. Examinations allow us to check side effects from treatment and whether they are resolving.

- Follow-up with certain tests (laboratory or imaging) that might detect a different cancer (we call these *secondary cancers* or *neoplasms*) as early as possible. The chances of these occurring depend on the treatment received. As an example, we worry about breast and lung cancers developing if we deliver radiation to the chest.

- Follow-up on cardiac function. Some patients receive chemotherapy that can damage the heart, so we occasionally do an echocardiogram (ultrasound of the heart) to check for any changes. Additionally, drugs such as doxorubicin (Adriamycin) can rarely cause heart failure.

- Follow-up tests on pulmonary function. Some of our treatments can damage the lung and cause fibrosis (like scarring). We might do pulmonary function tests at various intervals to evaluate. Again, drugs such as bleomycin can cause lung fibrosis.

- Blood work as part of routine examinations. This might detect early bone marrow function damage in situations where chemotherapy (especially at high doses) was given. We also check tumor markers when appropriate.

- Other tests that involve a discussion with the primary care physicians. Screening tests for different malignancies are still needed, but how they apply to a particular patient requires a discussion with their primary care doctor.

- Involving primary care doctors in some of the long-term issues. Hypertension, fertility, and sexual health are some examples where I relied heavily on my primary care colleagues to ensure patients received the best of care.

Other Issues

Patients deal with so many issues that are not directly related to physical or psychological complaints but can have a direct impact on both.

She asked me during our second visit after the diagnosis was confirmed and a treatment plan was being outlined: "Do I tell my children?"

She had a son and a daughter, both under the age of 10, and she had a form of lymphoma that would require six rounds of chemotherapy delivered every three weeks. One of the most common questions asked is how and when to inform family members, but children are unique in that there is fear over how the news might affect them emotionally.

CN: I think you should, but choose the right time. I have learned over the years that children are resilient, and having them support you during this journey helps you and them.

Patient: I don't want them to get sad.

CN: Some form of coping with an illness is OK and healthy. They will know something is up when you lose your hair, as this is expected. I think sitting down with them and discussing what is happening is the best strategy. Otherwise, they might be left to guess what is going on and could make up stories that are even scarier than the reality.

I have had patients who attempted to keep all illness issues private, and I think that might be doable for some time and with people who don't live with you. It is much harder when it comes to close relatives and people living with you. My recommendations have always been to inform close loved ones, relatives, and certainly members of your household. As a patient, you need that support system on this rocky road, and having them aware is going to enhance their ability to support you.

Relationships

Relationships vary from intimate to nonintimate, but a cancer diagnosis can change family dynamics. My advice is to be open and transparent, and to build a team around you as you navigate this new event. Your spouse, partner, children, or any other loved ones are likely scared and worried. They want to help and offer a hand, but they may be afraid of how that would be received, and they might not know how to help. No one is ever adequately prepared to care for someone diagnosed with cancer, so it is a new process for everyone involved. I have seen some relationships get much stronger because of a cancer diagnosis, but also some that were weakened and did not withstand the situation. Ensuring relationships survive a life-changing event such as cancer requires transparent communication. Choose the right time to discuss everything and anything from childcare (if applicable) to new feelings that may arise, sexual intimacy, and how social and daily routines might change. Sometimes, doctors or counselors can help foster this communication, but the most important consideration is to become a team.

Unfortunately, I have seen relationships dissipate in the face of cancer. Witnessing this was disheartening, but sometimes it was inevitable. I have relied on my counselors to help patients in these circumstances. My advice is to share what is happening in your life with the doctors. I will say that the biggest hurdle in relationships when cancer is diagnosed is communication. The more you communicate with your team and loved ones, the better the relationships will be across the board.

Work

The most common questions I have been asked by patients with cancer are:

- Do I tell my boss and coworkers?
- Do I need to change my work schedule? How?
- Now that I am done with treatment, can I return to work?

These are logical and important questions to address. I am from the school of thought that advocates for openness, even in the time of illness. This is important, so my advice has always been to call the human resources department and explain the situation. Your doctor can write a letter or a note if needed. Share with your direct supervisor the situation, as you might need to take some time off or take a leave of absence, or maybe take only intermittent time off when you need chemotherapy. The limitations need to be discussed with your oncologist, who might advise either against working full time or endorse continuing to work. I have recommended both based on the patient, the illness, the treatment, and the type of work.

When it comes to returning to work, sometimes the doctor might not allow it and may not be in favor. The decision depends on your mental and physical health, the demands of the job, the frequency of monitoring studies and follow-ups, and the type and severity of your symptoms. I am always in favor of patients returning to work even if it's part time because it gives them a sense of normalcy and purpose, but unfortunately, this is not always possible. Discussing with your doctor and with your HR personnel the Family and Medical Leave Act (FMLA) is important. FMLA applies to many workplaces, including private companies with at least 50 employees, and provides up to 12 weeks of unpaid time off for health reasons. FMLA leave may be taken in small increments, like hours or days. Also, limitations from cancer treatment are considered disabilities under the Americans with Disabilities Act (ADA), so employers must provide reasonable accommodations when needed.

My opinion is that sharing what you're going through with some select coworkers is reasonable, as this expands your support network and allows them to help you navigate the work environment and demands, similar to what your direct supervisor can do. It is always your choice not to share, but I have seen the upsides outweigh the downsides.

Finances

Cancer is an expensive disease. Patients might undergo several types of treatment (surgery, radiation, chemotherapy, targeted therapy, etc.), sometimes for an extended period. Moreover, patients might not be earning income, or their income is substantially less because they are not working full time. These problems weigh on patients and their loved ones as they are battling a serious disease. Instead of focusing on the disease and what needs to be done, they may be distracted by finances, which can lead to mental and physical anguish.

It is critical for doctors to screen for potential financial hardship the minute a cancer diagnosis is made. Screening should be repeated periodically as financial situations can change with time. The goal of screening is to identify high-risk patients for such hardship so that the medical team takes steps to mitigate these to the extent possible.

When hardship is recognized, the medical team might seek various avenues to help patients. My staff used to call foundations, patient-assistance programs at pharmaceutical companies, known philanthropists, hospital charity funds, or any organization that provides support services. The goal is to ensure that patients navigate this serious illness with as little stress on their finances as possible. Communicating your situation with your doctors and their staff is critical. There is help, and they know how to get it.

Many hospitals and cancer centers have invested in survivorship centers as physicians have recognized the medical and nonmedical issues facing cancer survivors. Addressing all of these is essential to improve overall survival of patients and their quality of life. These centers provide survivors with classes that span the spectrum of health, law, and finances. At one of the hospitals I worked at, we had a center that offered patients nutritional counseling, yoga and exercise classes, legal advice, financial counseling, and social work help. I believe that the trend will continue and expand as progress in cancer care is leading to more survivors. But with that, we must be attuned to their needs beyond simply the anticancer treatments.

Take-Home Points

- Survivorship in cancer starts from the time of a cancer diagnosis and lasts forever.

- Due to welcome medical advances, more patients survive cancer and are living. Currently, there are 18 million cancer survivors in the United States; that number was 3 million in 1971.

- Cancer survivors can suffer from various issues:

  - Psychological issues, such as anxiety, depression, survivor's guilt, and in extreme situations, suicidal ideations.

  - Physical issues, such as not maintaining muscle weight and suffering from persistent fatigue and lack of stamina.

  - Difficulty in managing employment issues, finances, and intimate relationships.

- Communicating about all things that affect the patient's daily living is critical. Doctors can help patients find resources needed, especially as there are more survivorship centers built across the United States. These can provide the additional resources survivors need.

CHAPTER 22

The Future of Cancer Care

My interest is in the future because
I am going to spend the rest of my life there.

—*Charles Kettering*

A Virtual World

It was May 2020, and my dad had an appointment with his cardiologist. As usual, he put on his nice clothes after a warm shower and even sprayed on some light cologne. We never left the house for the appointment as the world had shut down a few weeks earlier as a result of the COVID-19 pandemic; instead, we moved from the kitchen table to the living room. That was the extent of our commute to the cardiologist's clinic. After some computer hiccups, we finally saw the cardiologist's friendly face via an iPad screen, and he conducted the visit without listening to Dad's heart or lungs. He reviewed his medications; we discussed Dad's blood pressure, exercise program, and weight. The visit concluded.

Welcome to the virtual world of the healthcare system.

My dad was not thrilled with this—he craves human interaction and has always looked forward to meeting the clinical staff and communicating with them, despite his being hard of hearing. Personally, I was somewhat OK with it; I did not need to drive there and fight the traffic, and I saved time without cancelling any of my work meetings. But as a physician, I did not sense that my dad benefited much from that virtual visit. It was my perception, though; I could have been wrong.

Years after the emergency state of the pandemic has concluded, these virtual visits are still going strong. They are not as common, but they are part of the norm. In fact, one of my friends called me the other day to share that he had a virtual visit for a consultation regarding a benign growth that was removed off his back. He was given the choice of an in-person visit in six weeks or a virtual visit with the same doctor the following week. He chose the virtual route, reserving the in-person choice for later if needed. *Interesting*, I thought when he shared this with me, but it looks like this is mainstream now and is to be expected.

In the coming decade, I suspect there will be major changes not only in how we take care of patients and how well we understand science, but also in how we deliver care and how we conduct clinical trials.

The expansion of virtual platforms in health care, or what we call *telehealth*, is to be expected. I believe that many institutions will continue to offer the virtual option for some low-complexity follow-up care or even as an initial consultation for patients who live far away from the medical center. While some might have suspected that telehealth would be less common in oncology, as patients want to meet their oncologist face to face, I predict that it will become more of the norm in cancer care, but it will be for select, not all, patients. The virtual platform overcomes the challenges of distance and allows patients access to physicians that otherwise they wouldn't have had access to, and it can save time for all parties involved.

I envision that when doctors complete their visits, they will specify whether the return visits should be in person or virtual. Either option can be with the physician herself or with a member of the care team, such as a nurse or an advanced practice provider (APP). This distinction is a necessity as there are more patients who need to be seen than available hours at oncology practices, and many cancer centers want to reserve more time slots for new patients. I also believe that patients might want virtual options when they live far away, especially if their condition is stable. Now that insurance companies reimburse for telehealth, it is fair to assume that this service will continue expanding.

Another advantage of expanding the virtual platforms is that oncologists from low- and middle-income countries can access state-of-the-art physicians and academic progress. Patient cases can now be discussed across continents virtually, where oncologists from around the globe can review pathology and images at the click of a button. This provides indirect access to second opinions for patients who live thousands of miles away from specialized cancer centers.

Like anything, we must recognize that this technology has unintended consequences. Patients and their doctors must assert that virtual care does not replace in-person care but rather complements it for the betterment of the patient and in special circumstances.

Regulatory and Clinical Trials

More and more drugs will be approved by the FDA. This can be good as it accelerates patient access to potentially lifesaving therapies, but it's important to do so while ensuring a net benefit to patients. In other words, while we desire more and better drugs, these drugs must provide more benefit than harm and have manageable side effects.

The FDA is increasingly allowing manufacturers to bring drugs to market via an accelerated pathway. This pathway does not require the manufacturing company to conduct large studies and allows them to leverage surrogate endpoints and smaller phase 2 studies to show that their drugs indeed work. *Surrogate endpoints* are measures to assess whether a clinical trial is successful without relying on overall survival. The FDA defines surrogate endpoints in clinical trials as "indicators or signs used in place of another to tell if a treatment works." Surrogate endpoints include a shrinking tumor or lower biomarker levels. They may be used instead of stronger indicators, such as longer survival or improved quality of life, because the results of the smaller trial can be measured sooner. The increased use of surrogate endpoints in current and future clinical trials may allow earlier approval of new drugs to treat serious or life-threatening diseases, such as cancer. Surrogate endpoints, however, are not always true indicators of how well a treatment works unless confirmatory larger trials are conducted.

The law dictates that if a drug is approved via the accelerated pathway, the manufacturer must conduct a larger study that shows better survival or better quality of life. The FDA often works with manufacturers to guide them in how the trial must be designed so that the drug has the highest chance of getting the final traditional approval. The concern is that while we await the results of the larger trial, there is a chance that the drug being prescribed is not as good as we had hypothesized. Moreover, sometimes the FDA has occasionally not followed through in mandating the larger confirmatory trials. Finally, if the larger study fails to show the perceived benefit, we should reasonably expect that the drug gets withdrawn from the marketplace, but that does not always happen.

More drugs against cancer will be approved, and there will be an incremental need to educate physicians and patients about these drugs, their side effects, and their best positioning as anticancer therapies.

I also predict that most clinical trials investigating new anticancer therapies will explore oral drugs. More anticancer drugs are given by mouth now than ever before, and I suspect that this trend will continue, as it is perceived as easier for patients, and most of the novel "targeted" therapies are delivered orally.

When the COVID-19 pandemic hit the United States and the world, the FDA, investigators, manufacturers, and research organizations had to pivot to a virtual approach for conducting studies. Most clinical trials had strict inclusion and exclusion criteria dictating that patients had to undergo imaging and laboratory studies at the main site where the trial was open versus somewhere more convenient and local to the patient. That changed right away, and the FDA became more lenient on these practical elements. I am hoping that this continues as it never made sense to me that patients on studies needed to get their complete blood count (CBC) in my office versus a lab one block away from their house. We must put patients over bureaucracy.

It is fair to predict that we will increasingly use the virtual platforms and telehealth in how we conduct studies as long as we maintain guardrails to ensure patient safety and privacy.

From a regulatory perspective, I believe that there will be more use of real-world data (RWD) and evidence (RWE) to gain approvals of cancer drugs, especially as manufacturers increasingly use the accelerated approval pathway. I actually believe that this led to the launch of several big data companies across the globe helping manufacturers by providing them with RWD and RWE needed for the trials they are conducting.

RWD are data that are generated outside of clinical trials. Think of how much data there are outside of any clinical study. There are data on social media, pharmacy benefits, electronic health records, hospital records, insurance claims, and many more. The interest in RWD was heightened in December 2016 when the 21st Century Cures Act was enacted into law. The law is designed to "help accelerate medical product development and bring new innovations and advances to patients who need them faster and more efficiently." It has been well known that few patients in the United States are treated on trials and that most patients are treated in a real-world setting. Understanding the inherent differences between trial and real-world patient characteristics is important, and the FDA has recognized that. Therefore, they have encouraged manufacturers to use RWD for some regulatory approvals as long as the data sources and the real-world study are discussed with the FDA so that all parties agree on the deliverables and endpoints.

The Cures Act also "defined clinical outcome assessment" as a measurement of symptoms, mental state, and effect of treatment on patient functions, but it also included patient-reported outcomes, or PROs; "these are measures of a patient's health status as reported directly from the patient without added interpretation by a healthcare worker or anyone else, such as a pain scale."

The main challenge was how to get the PROs in an efficient manner since our routine clinical care means that physicians ask patients how they feel when they do the "review of systems," or ROS. The ROS process, however, has its own limitations as physicians might focus on the side effects *they* think are important while patients might be concerned about something completely different. It's like asking a patient about headaches and focusing on that symptom because it is what predicted the type of therapy the patient is on, but the patient is more concerned about their constipation.

I predict that with time, we will be implementing PROs more frequently in routine clinical trials and certainly in most large clinical trials. In 2017, Dr. Basch showed that incorporating PROs metrics and measures as part of clinical care can lead to better survival for patients with cancer. The reason PROs have not been widely used is simply logistics and the fact that not all oncologists have embraced their importance, since doctors "know better" what side effects to look for—a notion I never agreed with.

No one knows what bothers or helps a patient more than the patient does. PROs embody that concept and will continue to do so. Manufacturers understand now that PROs are needed as part of their regulatory trials, and they have started looking at various ways to capture those data moving forward.

Healthcare Delivery

When I think of healthcare delivery, I think of payers (government and commercial insurance companies) and healthcare providers. Other stakeholders are very important, but these two are essential as payers dictate what medications we can prescribe, and providers decide what drugs are indeed prescribed.

Payers will face exponentially expensive cancer drugs, and how these are covered will become increasingly challenging. How cancer drugs are paid for is beyond the scope of this book and can be a book by itself. But it is worth noting that the Inflation Reduction Act, passed in 2022, allows the government to negotiate prices of some drugs, including cancer drugs, based on their cost. That won't begin until 2026 and is limited to 10 drugs for now, not all of which are oncology ones. The impact of that law on healthcare cost overall will not be known for years to come. As more drugs with similar mechanisms and indications make it into the oncology market, I predict that payers will increasingly use RWD to better understand how these drugs are prescribed and whether the cost of care is higher with one versus another.

Let me illustrate. Imagine drugs A and B are indicated for the same cancer at the same stage and they have similar mechanisms of action, but they are manufactured by two different pharmaceutical companies. It is fair to say that both companies would want their drug to capture a higher market share. To do so, manufacturers can negotiate with payers various rebates that could save the payer dollars in exchange for making their drug the preferred one. In these negotiations, manufacturers often need to demonstrate that their drug can save cost to the payer, and they often leverage RWD to prove that when patients take their drug, they are less likely to be hospitalized or go to the ER. Manufacturers also use RWD to show that adherence to their respective drugs is better than the competition's, a metric that is appealing to payers as it can reduce ER visits.

Moving forward, I suspect payers will be more critical of RWD so that they decide strategically how to cover the cost of these drugs. Payers realize that clinical trial patients are highly selective and not always representative of the real world. This is why manufacturers are attempting to be more pragmatic in their clinical studies and more inclusive of patients who represent the real world. This allows manufacturers to leverage their data—when available—in their negotiation with payers, arguing that their drugs have shown utility and benefit in similar demographics to those in routine clinical practices.

From the provider's perspective, oncologists are also being scrutinized to deliver cost-effective therapies. There have been various models to guide oncologists in how best to do so, and whether these have been successful remains to be seen. While payers often dictate what oncologists can prescribe, large oncology networks have been successful in executing on shared-saving contracts with local, regional, or national payers. The essence of these is that prescribers adhere to certain agreed-on metrics, and if these are achieved, oncologists can share a percentage of the savings with payers. It is viewed as a win-win scenario. From a payer's side, they can save money by demanding reasonable metrics, such as no chemotherapy in the last two weeks of life or discussing "do not resuscitate" (DNR) status within two or three oncology visits. From the provider's perspective, the win is a reasonable financial incentive as long as the metrics are supported by evidence and are patient centric.

Oncologists will continuously be asked to be cognizant of the cost of their cancer care delivery; however, many practices have also been struggling to stay afloat and solvent from a revenue perspective. I predict that more community oncology practices will either merge with each other or will be acquired by large healthcare systems or academic institutions. It is rather inevitable, but I do fear that this might limit available choices for patients. I am a believer that with more choices, patients are served best. I also believe that community practices will continue to seek additional revenue streams as their profit margins shrink. To that end, many oncologists would want to own their own imaging centers and would consider joint ventures with radiation oncology centers so that patients can stay within their system versus going away to larger hospitals or universities.

Moreover, with increased demand for oncologists, more utilization of advanced practice providers (APPs) has taken place. These are either nurse practitioners (NPs) or physician assistants (PAs) who have advanced training and can help care for patients with cancer. Within their scope, they can prescribe drugs and have become an integral component of the cancer care delivery system. I predict that APPs will become even more important in all aspects of cancer care delivery, and how they are used might vary among centers and practices. Most, however, use APPs in follow-up visits, lower-complexity patients, survivorship clinics, toxicity assessment visits, and assistance with procedures such as bone marrow biopsies or lumbar punctures. This allows more time for oncologists to see new patients and potentially reduce wait times. My prediction is that more APPs will enter the oncology space, and more patients will be seen by APPs for their routine oncology care.

Artificial Intelligence (AI)

In simple terms, artificial intelligence means that computers and machines help us either diagnose complex problems or decide how best to treat a patient. I don't think we can give AI justice in this book, but I predict that we will use large sets of patients' clinical and molecular data to help us potentially deliver better care.

I recorded a few podcasts on this topic, and after each one, I scratched my head even more. I needed to resolve and simplify where AI could best help, as some physicians have become concerned that their jobs may be in jeopardy because computers might take over. The reality is that computers and machines will aid doctors, not replace them. As a practicing oncologist, I would want AI to help me in challenging oncology situations.

Several areas in oncology can benefit from AI. As an example, in radiology (and I am not a radiologist), I can imagine that some imaging studies show abnormalities that are tough to interpret but may be suspicious of cancer. Maybe AI can help predict the likelihood that such findings are serious so we can determine whether a biopsy is needed. Avoiding unnecessary biopsies can reduce complications and cost, which is definitely the right thing to do for patients.

Another area that may benefit is pathology. Maybe AI can help differentiate difficult pathological findings to provide a more accurate diagnosis. I can envision a future where applying AI on digitized pathology images can aid pathologists and oncologists in determining which molecular mutation is most likely in a particular patient.

I can also see the value in AI helping us to build algorithms that might optimize how we treat patients. Imagine a disease that has various treatment options, and which regimen is chosen is often empiric. I can see AI being applied to large datasets that have looked at various treatment options in this particular disease, and through various data mining strategies, the output can guide physicians in treatment selection or deciding the proper sequence of treatment.

Maybe AI can assist in generating algorithms that help physicians know beforehand which of their patients is at highest risk if being admitted to the hospital based on available electronic medical record data. Armed with this information, physicians can take measures to mitigate such a possibility.

The principle in any AI-based process is that we train machines to interpret data, but success depends on the level of data we enter and its accuracy. With that said, being critical of data remains the rate-limiting step for the success of AI.

There is some potential for AI to help diagnose and treat cancer, but the jury is still out on how and whether it will improve the work real people do.

Precision Oncology

As physicians, we pride ourselves on treating patients with the right medicine at the right time with the right dose. It's the essence of medicine beyond oncology; isn't treating an infection with the right antibiotics for the correct duration and with the right dose considered precision medicine? But in oncology, this precise approach to treating cancer has taken on a different color. It implies that we are targeting the exact genes that drive cancer cell growth.

My first glimpse of the power of precision oncology came to light when I was a fellow at Northwestern University and was helping enroll CML patients on the original imatinib trial I mentioned in prior chapters. The responses I witnessed were dramatic. As I discussed earlier, CML cells have the pathognomonic (9;22) chromosomal translocation that leads to producing an abnormal protein, which imatinib targets, thus killing the leukemia cells.

There are so many similar examples in oncology, but their underpinning is knowing what drives the cancer, then developing drugs that can target that "driver."

I believe the knowledge of the mutations that drive some cancers' development was enhanced as the human genome was sequenced. This means that scientists were able to identify the composition of the human genome. By knowing what is normal in the genome, we can identify what's not. We can then attack the abnormal areas that might be contributing to cancer development with drugs designed against these specific abnormalities.

How did we know the human genome composition? This was done using a technique called *DNA sequencing.* It is the understanding of the blocks that bind together to form the DNA and their sequence.

DNA sequencing means using technology to determine the order of the four chemical building blocks that make the DNA (we call these *bases,* as you know from chapter 1). The sequence explains the genetic information carried on every DNA segment, which can lead to turning some genes on, turning other genes off, and causing other genetic changes that may be involved in causing cancers or other diseases.

Back in the early 2000s, the sequencing technology was not advanced; it was also cumbersome and expensive. This has changed to where the entire genome of a patient can be sequenced for just a few thousand dollars—not to say that this is cheap, but it's certainly much cheaper and easier to do than it was 20 years ago. The method by which DNA is sequenced has evolved and advanced in various ways, all of which led to the completion of the Human Genome Project in 2003. This sequencing process is known in the medical field as *next-generation sequencing*, or NGS. And it has gone through various advances, leading to better sensitivity, cheaper cost, high throughput, and faster results.

NGS allows us to identify abnormalities in the sequence that lead to mutations, and we can tell if these mutations are somatic (acquired) or germline (inherited). If we are sequencing the DNA, we call this *DNAseq*, and if we are sequencing the RNA, we call this *RNAseq*. As you know by now, the ultimate product of DNA is protein, so if the sequence of the DNA blocks is altered, we might end up with the wrong protein that could lead to evolution of disease, including cancer. Think of this as having the correct digits to a phone number. If one number is misplaced, you'll dial the wrong number. If the DNA building blocks are not organized in the proper manner, the wrong protein will develop. The wrong number gets you the wrong person, and the wrong protein potentially gets you a disease. The good news is that our bodies are resilient and can repair many damages in these blocks—but sometimes we can't.

The most commonly used form of NGS is *whole-genome sequencing* (WGS), where we analyze the entire sequence across the entire genome. *Whole-exome sequencing* (WES) refers to sequencing only the areas involved in building the protein. In other words, we are really interested in the meat and not the fluff. In real life, WES is what matters as we can look at the blocks that are crucial versus the ones that are just there and are not involved in any protein manufacturing. Only 2% of the genome represents the regions that code for proteins. Due to the reduced sequencing burden, WES can also offer a more cost-effective option than WGS and reduce the volume and complexity of the resultant sequencing data. By sequencing only a fraction of the genome, however, vital information may be missed and the opportunity for novel discoveries is reduced. Many contend that WGS, therefore, offers a more powerful analysis that can reveal a more complete picture.

With more patients undergoing NGS, doctors can determine what is driving the growth and development of some cancers. This in turns leads to making drugs that specifically target the particular driver of a cancer, if known. This is what we mean by precision oncology in the modern era. It is beyond treating the right patient with the right drug at the right time with the right dose; rather, it is treating the exact genetic mutation that we know led to that cancer. Of course, this assumes that we know what mutations drive all cancers (we don't) and that we have drugs against any mutation we might detect (we don't). But this does not mean that we might not in the future. There have been many advances, and we have more targets and more drugs than ever before.

What if we find several mutations? Sometimes they all work together to transform the cells into cancerous ones, but at times, one of these mutations is the real "driver," while another can be a "bystander." Only through research can we determine whether what we find is a true signal or noise.

I recall attending a lecture by a major scientist who spent his life studying an oncogene called *K-RAS*. The conclusion of his studies was that when this oncogene was present, the cancer became aggressive, and that *K-RAS* was a target that we could never develop a drug against. Fast-forward to today, and we have drugs that specifically target *K-RAS* and are able to control the growth of some cancers that are driven by it.

Many advanced cancers now undergo NGS so that doctors can understand their molecular building blocks, but not all patients who qualify for this technology indeed undergo it. Barriers to NGS vary from educational gaps in which doctors don't understand its rational and cannot interpret the results, to patients being concerned about undergoing any molecular studies due to data privacy concerns. NGS is also being studied at much earlier stages of the cancers, and treatment at times is determined by the results. An example is the lung cancer that is driven by the *EGFR* mutation. After surgery for early-stage disease, patients who carry that mutation benefit from three years of osimertinib, a drug that targets the *EGFR* mutation and improves survival for these patients.

In the years to come, there will be more advances in precision oncology. The underpinning of this concept is the fact that somatic mutations are the foundation of cancer development, so we need to identify them, and the best way to do so is through NGS.

In addition to testing these mutations by "sequencing" the cancer tissue, advances are being made to sequence the blood in cancer patients to detect the tumor cell DNA and/or RNA. This is called *liquid biopsy*. The concept is that tumors shed their cells into the blood and that scientific assays can detect these cells accurately. Liquid biopsies have gained popularity in recent years, as there are situations where biopsying the actual tissue can be challenging for various reasons.

Liquid biopsies allow physicians to check for *minimal residual disease* (MRD), which is basically detecting a tumor on the molecular level before we can see it on imaging studies. The idea is that by doing so, we can predict patients at highest risk of relapse and potentially can intervene earlier. As an example, think of a patient with colon cancer who has undergone surgery. We can envision a scenario whereby checking MRD shows that there are cells in the blood related to the disease, and maybe giving that patient treatment can help prevent the cancer from coming back. On the other hand, withholding treatment in someone like this patient who has MRD-negative blood might be reasonable and avoids toxicities of chemotherapy that otherwise would have been administered. Today, the scientific world is not completely ready to not treat a cancer patient who is MRD negative, but I can envision a future state where this might be the case.

Also, the availability of liquid biopsies is allowing some companies to work on what we call *multicancer early detection* (MCED), a hypothesis that allows doctors to potentially assess the likelihood of healthy people developing various cancers by simply doing such a blood test. It is not clear whether this is recommended for all people or just people at high risk of developing certain cancers, but research continues to evaluate whether MCED testing is something doctors should recommend. Some tests are being advertised directly to the consumer, and that might be a bit problematic as I personally view MCED the way I view any screening test (see chapter 2); therefore, supervising the decision and output by a knowledgeable healthcare professional is ideal.

Knowing the molecular mechanisms of certain cancers has also allowed the development of CRISPR technology. Simply put, this is gene editing, meaning that we are modifying the genes that we know have affected the development of disease, including cancer. There are different ways to edit the genome, all beyond this text, but it is exciting to start thinking of modifying the essence of why a cancer has developed. As this book goes to press, two therapies have been approved by the FDA to treat sickle cell disease using CRISPR technology.

Tumor-Agnostic Therapies

Some mutations can be found in different cancers from different organs. Think of a breast cancer and a pancreatic cancer that both have the same molecular foundation that might have led to their development. The idea of a "tumor agnostic therapy" is to deliver a drug that treats the cancer based on the cancer's genetics and molecular features, regardless of the cancer type or which part of the body it started from.

I still think the origin of the tumor matters as there are elements of the "host" environment that might make a difference and lead to either better response or more resistance to therapy, but I do predict that more and more drugs will be approved regardless of where the tumor had originated. These drugs are called *tissue-agnostic* or *tumor-agnostic* drugs because they can be used for various cancers.

I know that some other types of traditional chemotherapy drugs are used for different cancers regardless of their location, but we don't call these tumor-agnostic because they are not developed based on the molecular features and underpinnings of the tumor. I thought I'd provide a quick list of these tumor-agnostic drugs:

Pembrolizumab (Keytruda): Pembrolizumab is approved for use in any cancer that has a deficiency in genes called *mismatch repair genes* or tumors that have "high microsatellite instability," as well as in tumors that have high tumor mutational burden. These are tumors that have frequent genetic mutations. I discuss immunotherapy drugs in chapter 14.

Larotrectinib (Vitrakvi): Some cancer cells have mutations in one of the *NTRK* genes that lead to cancer cell growth. Larotrectinib is an oral drug given for tumors that have that mutation, regardless of which organ they originated from.

Entrectinib (Rozlytrek): This too targets the *NTRK* gene, but it was also found to help lung cancer patients who carry an abnormal *ROS1* gene.

Dostarlimab (Jemperli): This form of immunotherapy blocks PD-1 and can be used when there are defects in a mismatch repair gene.

Dabrafenib and trametinib (Tafinlar and Mekinist): The first targets the BRAF protein and the second targets the MEK protein. They are used when a patients with solid tumors who have a genetic mutation called *BRAF* V600E. This is evidence that the location of the cancer cells still matters even when we know the molecular features of the tumor.

Selpercatinib (Retevmo): This drug targets tumors that carry mutations in the *RET* gene, leading to an abnormal RET protein.

In the years to come, more patients will undergo NGS, and we will have a better idea of what might have driven their cells to become cancerous. In knowing this, the hope is to be more precise in deciding what therapy to give, which could lead to better outcomes, fewer side effects, and lower cost of care. Drug manufacturers will also be smarter in deciding which targets they need to develop drugs against, allowing them to become more strategic.

Take-Home Points

- The future of cancer care is bright. We know more about cancer than ever, and we have better drugs than we ever could have imagined.

- More patients will have access to telehealth, and more artificial intelligence (AI) applications will be used in cancer care.

- There will be an increased role for advanced practice providers (APPs) in cancer care delivery.

- There will be more mergers and acquisitions among healthcare systems.

- There will be more flexibility in clinical trials due to some remote capabilities being embraced.

- More drugs will be approved using accelerated pathways and surrogate endpoints.

- More newly approved cancer drugs are likely to be oral therapies.

- More real-word-data (RWD) and real-world-evidence (RWE) studies will be conducted, and more of these will be used for regulatory approvals.

- Next-generation sequencing (NGS) will become routine in all advanced cancers and in most early-stage cancer.

- Almost all cancer patients will undergo germline testing to check for hereditary genes.

- More patients will survive these cancers, and we will continue to wage—and often win—the war against this disease.

Acknowledgments

This book was a dream come true. It has been a privilege to walk alongside hundreds of patients as they have progressed through their cancer journey. To be able to then take those experiences and express them in words is a cherished honor. This dream could not have been realized without the support and encouragement of my loving family, who tolerated (once again) my long hours typing at coffee shops all over the Chicagoland area. My deepest gratitude, thanks, and love to my wife Lama; my sons Yazan and Zane; my wonderful parents, whose unconditional love is the biggest prize I have in life; my brother Fadi and his family; my amazing loving sister Dina; and all my friends and loved ones who encouraged me to write this book and believed that I could do it, even when I doubted myself.

I want to thank my patients, who have trusted me throughout my career with their care. I hope I never failed you, and I hope you all know that I cared about each one of you like a member of my own family. I always gave 100% and did my best. Sometimes I succeeded, while other times I failed; please know that each one of you taught me something about life and living. Without you and the stories you shared with me, this book could not have been possible.

My deepest and sincerest thanks to Johns Hopkins University Press, who believed in me and stood behind this book as my esteemed publisher. Special thanks to Alena Jones and Suzanne Staszak-Silva, who worked with me to make this book the real piece you hold in your hands today. I am grateful to them, and to all other staff members at the Press.

Special thanks to Dr. Sandeep Parsad from the University of Chicago, who read a few chapters of this book when it was incepted and provided valuable and amazing feedback that allowed me to better refine the messaging. Thank you to my friend and colleague Dr. Salma Jabbour from Rutgers Cancer Institute, who provided valuable feedback on the radiation therapy chapter.

Thank you to everyone I read a few excerpts to and who told me to keep going, even when I was in doubt. I hope you all know how grateful I am.

And thank you to all the oncologists, researchers, scientists, and everyone who works to help patients with cancer. Patients are forever grateful to the advances in science, and I thank you on their behalf.

Sources

CHAPTER 1

1. Elmore, Susan. 2007. "Apoptosis: A Review of Programmed Cell Death." *Toxic Pathology* 35(4): 495–516. https://doi.org/10.1080/01926230701320337.

2. De, S., and S. Ganesan. 2017. "Looking beyond Drivers and Passengers in Cancer Genome Sequencing Data." *Annals of Oncology* 28(5): 938–45. https://doi.org/10.1093/annonc/mdw677.

3. Kasisomayajula, Viswanath, Roy S. Herbst, Stephanie R. Land, Scott J. Leischow, Peter G. Shields, Thomas H. Brandon, Michael C. Fiore, et al. 2010. "Tobacco and Cancer: An American Association for Cancer Research Policy Statement." *Cancer Research* 70(9): 3419–30. https://doi.org/10.1158/0008-5472.CAN-10-1087.

4. Rumgay, Harriet, Neil Murphy, Pietro Ferrari, and Isabelle Soerjomataram. 2021. "Alcohol and Cancer: Epidemiology and Biological Mechanisms." *Nutrients* 13(9): 3173–87. https://doi.org/10.3390/nu13093173.

5. Sung, Hyuna, Rebecca L. Siegel, Philip S. Rosenberg, and Ahmedin Jemal. 2019. "Emerging Cancer Trends among Young Adults in the USA: Analysis of a Population-Based Cancer Registry." *Lancet Public Health* 4(3): e137–47. https://doi.org/10.1016/S2468-2667(18)30267-6.

6. Green, Eric. 2023. "Gene." National Human Genome Research Institute. https://www.genome.gov/genetics-glossary/Gene.

7. National Cancer Institute. 2021. "What Is Cancer?" https://www.cancer.gov/about-cancer/understanding/what-is-cancer.

8. National Human Genome Research Institute. 2023. "Apoptosis." National Institutes of Health. https://www.genome.gov/genetics-glossary/apoptosis.

9. American Cancer Society. n.d. "Cancer Risk and Prevention." https://www
.cancer.org/healthy/cancer-causes.html. Accessed Nov. 11, 2023.

10. American Cancer Society. 2019. "Ultraviolet Radiation." https://www
.cancer.org/cancer/risk-prevention/sun-and-uv/uv-radiation.html.

11. The University of Texas MD Anderson Cancer Center. 2018. "7 Viruses
That Cause Cancer." https://www.mdanderson.org/publications/focused
-on-health/7-viruses-that-cause-cancer.h17-1592202.html.

12. McDowell, Sandy. 2021. "Smoking Rates Historically Low, but Other
Cancer-Related Behaviors Need Improvement." https://www.cancer.org
/research/acs-research-news/acs-report-smoking-rates-historically-low
-but-other-cancer-related-behaviors-need-improvement.html.

13. National Cancer Institute. 2021. "Alcohol and Cancer Risk." https://www
.cancer.gov/about-cancer/causes-prevention/risk/alcohol/alcohol-fact-sheet.

CHAPTER 2

1. US Preventive Services Task Force. 2016. "Breast Cancer: Screening."
https://www.uspreventiveservicestaskforce.org/uspstf/recommendation
/breast-cancer-screening.

2. Breastcancer.org. 2022. "Breast MRI (Magnetic Resonance Imaging)."
https://www.breastcancer.org/symptoms/testing/types/mri/screening.

3. Ratini, Melinda. 2022. "What Is Tomosynthesis for Breast Cancer
Diagnosis?" https://www.webmd.com/breast-cancer/guide/tomosynthesis
-breast-cancer.

4. Centers for Disease Control and Prevention. 2023. "What Should I Know
about Screening?" https://www.cdc.gov/cancer/colorectal/basic_info
/screening/index.htm.

5. Bretthauer, Michael, Magnus Loberg, Paulina Wieszczy, Mette Kalager,
Louise Emilsson, Kjetil Garborg, Maciej Rupinski, et al. 2022. "Effect of
Colonoscopy Screening on Risks of Colorectal Cancer and Related Death."
New England Journal of Medicine 387(17): 1547–56. https://doi.org/10.1056
/NEJMoa2208375.

6. National Cancer Institute. 2023. "Cervical Cancer Screening." https://
www.cancer.gov/types/cervical/pap-hpv-testing-fact-sheet.

7. US Preventive Services Task Force. 2018. "Cervical Cancer: Screening." https://www.uspreventiveservicestaskforce.org/uspstf/recommendation/cervical-cancer-screening.

8. Cheng, Liqin, Yan Wang, and Juan Du. 2020. "Human Papillomavirus Vaccines: An Updated Review." *Vaccines* 8(3): 391–411. https://doi.org/10.3390/vaccines8030391.

9. National Cancer Institute. 2023. "Prostate Cancer Screening (PDQ®)–Patient Version." https://www.cancer.gov/types/prostate/patient/prostate-screening-pdq. Accessed Nov. 11, 2023.

10. Anderiole, Gerald L., E. David Crawford, Robert L. Grubb III, Saundra S. Buys, David Chia, Timothy R. Church, Mona N. Fouad, et al. 2009. "Mortality Results from a Randomized Prostate-Cancer Screening Trial." *New England Journal of Medicine* 360(13): 1310–19. https://doi.org/10.1056/NEJMoa0810696.

11. Schroder, Fritz H., Jonas Hugosson, Monique J. Roobol, Teuvo L. J. Tammela, Stefano Ciatto, Vera Nelen, Maciej Kwiatkowski, et al. 2009. "Screening and Prostate-Cancer Mortality in a Randomized European Study." *New England Journal of Medicine* 360(13): 1320–28. https://doi.org/10.1056/NEJMoa0810084.

12. National Cancer Institute. 2023. "Lung Cancer Screening (PDQ®)–Patient Version." https://www.cancer.gov/types/lung/patient/lung-screening-pdq.

13. National Cancer Institute. n.d. "Patient and Physician Guide: National Lung Screening Trial." https://www.cancer.gov/types/lung/research/nlst studyguidepatientsphysicians.pdf. Accessed Nov. 11, 2023.

14. The National Lung Screening Trial Research Team. 2011. "Reduced Lung-Cancer Mortality with Low-Dose Computed Tomographic Screening." *New England Journal of Medicine* 365(5): 395–409. https://doi.org/10.1056/NEJMoa1102873.

15. de Koning, Harry J., Carlijn M. van der Aalst, Pim A. de Jong, Ernst T. Scholten, Kristiaan Nackaerts, Marjolein A. Heuvelmans, Jan-Willem J. Lammers, et al. 2020. "Reduced Lung-Cancer Mortality with Volume CT Screening in a Randomized Trial." *New England Journal of Medicine* 382(6): 503–13. https://doi.org/10.1056/NEJMoa1911793.

16. Jonas, Daniel E., Daniel S. Reuland, Shivani M. Reddy, Max Nagle, Stephen D. Clark, Rachel Palmieri Weber, Chineme Enyioha, et al. 2021. "Screening for Lung Cancer with Low-Dose Computed Tomography: Updated Evidence Report and Systematic Review for the US Preventive Services Task Force." *JAMA* 325(10): 971–87. https://doi.org/10.1001/jama.2021.0377.

17. National Cancer Institute. 2023. "Skin Cancer Screening (PDQ®)–Patient Version." https://www.cancer.gov/types/skin/patient/skin-screening-pdq.

CHAPTER 3

1. American Cancer Society. 2020. "Signs and Symptoms of Cancer." https://www.cancer.org/treatment/understanding-your-diagnosis/signs-and-symptoms-of-cancer.html.

2. Cancer Research UK. 2022. "Signs and Symptoms of Cancer." https://www.cancerresearchuk.org/about-cancer/cancer-symptoms.

CHAPTER 4

1. American Society of Clinical Oncology. 2021. "Biopsy." Cancer.Net. https://www.cancer.net/navigating-cancer-care/diagnosing-cancer/tests-and-procedures/biopsy.

2. Hamilton, William. 2010. "Cancer Diagnosis in Primary Care." *British Journal of General Practice* 60(571): 121–28. https://doi.org/10.3399/bjgp10X483175.

3. National Cancer Institute. 2023. "How Cancer Is Diagnosed." https://www.cancer.gov/about-cancer/diagnosis-staging/diagnosis. Accessed Nov. 11, 2023.

4. College of American Pathologists. n.d. "What Is Pathology?" https://www.cap.org/member-resources/articles/what-is-pathology. Accessed Dec. 22, 2023.

CHAPTER 6

1. American College of Surgeons. n.d. "Cancer Staging Systems." https://www.facs.org/quality-programs/cancer-programs/american-joint-committee-on-cancer/cancer-staging-systems/. Accessed Nov. 11, 2023.

2. National Cancer Institute. 2022. "Cancer Staging." https://www.cancer
    .gov/about-cancer/diagnosis-staging/staging.

CHAPTER 7

1. Olver, Ian, Mariko Carey, Jamie Bryant, Allison Boyes, Tiffany Evans, and
    Rob Sanson-Fisher. 2020. "Second Opinions in Medical Oncology." *BMC
    Palliative Care* 19(1): 112–20. https://doi.org/10.1186/s12904-020-00619-9.

2. Hillen, Marji A., Niki M. Medendorp, Joost G. Daams, and Ellen M. A.
    Smets. 2017. "Patient-Driven Second Opinions in Oncology: A Systematic
    Review." *Oncologist* 22(10): 1197–211. https://doi.org/10.1634/theoncol
    ogist.2016-0429.

CHAPTER 8

1. McKinney, Mishellene, Rose Bell, Cindy Samborski, Kristopher At-
    wood, Grace Dean, Katherine Eakle, and Stephen Edge. 2021. "Clinical
    Trial Participation: A Pilot Study of Patient-Identified Barriers." *Clinical
    Journal of Oncology Nursing* 25(6): 647–54. https://doi.org/10.1188/21.cjon
    .647-654.

2. Grants and Funding. n.d. "NIH's Definition of a Clinical Trial." National
    Institutes of Health. https://grants.nih.gov/policy/clinical-trials/definition
    .htm. Accessed Dec. 23, 2023.

3. Stark, Laura, and Jeremy A. Greene. 2016. "Clinical Trials, Healthy Con-
    trols, and the Birth of the IRB." *New England Journal of Medicine* 375(11):
    1013–15. https://doi.org/10.1056/nejmp1607653.

4. Bothwell, Laura E., and Scott H. Podolsky. 2016. "The Emergence of the
    Randomized, Controlled Trial." *New England Journal of Medicine* 375(6):
    501–4. https://doi.org/10.1056/nejmp1604635.

5. Grady, Christine, Steven R. Cummings, Michael C. Rowbotham, Mi-
    chael V. McConnell, Euan A. Ashley, and Gagandeep Kang. 2017. "In-
    formed Consent." Edited by Jeffrey M. Drazen, David P. Harrington,
    John J. V. McMurray, James H. Ware, and Janet Woodcock. *New England
    Journal of Medicine* 376(9): 856–67. https://doi.org/10.1056/nejmra1603773.

6. Ford, Ian, and John Norrie. 2016. "Pragmatic Trials." Edited by Jeffrey M.
    Drazen, David P. Harrington, John J. V. McMurray, James H. Ware, and

Janet Woodcock. *New England Journal of Medicine* 375(5): 454–63. https://doi.org/10.1056/nejmra1510059.

7. National Institute on Aging. 2023. "What Are Clinical Trials and Studies?" National Institutes of Health. https://www.nia.nih.gov/health/what-are-clinical-trials-and-studies. Accessed Nov. 12, 2023.

8. National Library of Medicine. 2019. "Learn about Studies." ClinicalTrials.gov. 2019. https://clinicaltrials.gov/study-basics/learn-about-studies.

9. Adashek, Jacob J., Patricia M. LoRusso, David S. Hong, and Razelle Kurzrock. 2019. "Phase I Trials as Valid Therapeutic Options for Patients with Cancer." *Nature Reviews Clinical Oncology* 16(12): 773–78. https://doi.org/10.1038/s41571-019-0262-9.

10. Ivy, S. Percy, Lillian L. Siu, Elizabeth Garrett-Mayer, and Larry Rubinstein. 2010. "Approaches to Phase 1 Clinical Trial Design Focused on Safety, Efficiency, and Selected Patient Populations: A Report from the Clinical Trial Design Task Force of the National Cancer Institute Investigational Drug Steering Committee." *Clinical Cancer Research* 16(6): 1726–36. https://doi.org/10.1158/1078-0432.CCR-09-1961.

11. Brown, S. R., W. M. Gregory, C. J. Twelves, M. Buyse, F. Collinson, M. Parmar, M. T. Seymour, and J. M. Brown. 2011. "Designing Phase II Trials in Cancer: A Systematic Review and Guidance." *British Journal of Cancer* 105(2): 194–99. https://doi.org/10.1038/bjc.2011.235.

12. American Cancer Society. 2020. "Types and Phases of Clinical Trials." https://www.cancer.org/treatment/treatments-and-side-effects/clinical-trials/what-you-need-to-know/phases-of-clinical-trials.html.

13. Druker, Brian J., Moshe Talpaz, Debra J. Resta, Bin Peng, Elisabeth Buchdunger, John M. Ford, Nicholas B. Lydon, et al. 2001. "Efficacy and Safety of a Specific Inhibitor of the BCR-ABL Tyrosine Kinase in Chronic Myeloid Leukemia." *New England Journal of Medicine* 344: 1031–37. https://www.nejm.org/doi/full/10.1056/nejm200104053441401.

14. US Department of Health and Human Services. 1979. *The Belmont Report: Ethical Principles and Guidelines for the Protection of Human Subjects of Research.* Washington, DC: Department of Health, Education, and Welfare. https://www.hhs.gov/ohrp/regulations-and-policy/belmont-report/read-the-belmont-report/index.html.

CHAPTER 9

1. Lamb, B., J. S. A. Green, C. Vincent, and N. Sevdalis. 2011. "Decision Making in Surgical Oncology." *Surgical Oncology* 20(3): 163–68. https://doi .org/10.1016/j.suronc.2010.07.007.

2. Bakalar, Nicholas. 2021. "Are Robotic Surgeries Really Better?" *New York Times*, August 16, 2021, sec. Well. https://www.nytimes.com/2021/08/16 /well/live/robotic-surgery-benefits.html.

3. American Society of Clinical Oncology. 2023. "What Is Cancer Surgery?" Cancer.Net. https://www.cancer.net/navigating-cancer-care/how-cancer -treated/surgery/what-cancer-surgery. Accessed Nov. 12, 2023.

4. National Cancer Institute. 2015. "Surgery to Treat Cancer." https://www .cancer.gov/about-cancer/treatment/types/surgery.

5. Berlinger, Norman T. 2006. "Robotic Surgery—Squeezing into Tight Places." *New England Journal of Medicine* 354(20): 2099–101. https://doi.org /10.1056/nejmp058233.

6. Cohen, Joshua T., and Thomas J. Miner. 2021. "Who Should Decide When Palliative Surgery Is Justifiable?" *AMA Journal of Ethics* 23(10): 761–65. https://doi.org/10.1001/amajethics.2021.761.

7. Deo, S. V. S., Naveen Kumar, Vinaya Kumar J. Rajendra, Sunil Kumar, Sandeep Kumar Bhoriwal, Mukurdipi Ray, Sushma Bhatnagar, and Seema Mishra. 2021. "Palliative Surgery for Advanced Cancer: Clinical Profile, Spectrum of Surgery and Outcomes from a Tertiary Care Cancer Centre in Low-Middle-Income Country." *Indian Journal of Palliative Care* 27(2): 281–85. https://doi.org/10.25259/ijpc_399_20.

8. Simillis, Constantinos, Nikhil Lal, Sarah N. Thoukididou, Christos Kontovounisios, Jason J. Smith, Roel Hompes, Michel Adamina, and Paris P. Tekkis. 2019. "Open versus Laparoscopic versus Robotic versus Transanal Mesorectal Excision for Rectal Cancer." *Annals of Surgery* 270(1): 59–68. https://doi.org/10.1097/sla.0000000000003227.

9. Bramhe, Sakshi, and Swanand S. Pathak. 2022. "Robotic Surgery: A Narra- tive Review." *Cureus* 14(9): e29179. https://doi.org/10.7759/cureus.29179.

10. Sayari, Arash J., Coralie Pardo, Bryce A. Basques, and Matthew W. Colman. 2019. "Review of Robotic-Assisted Surgery: What the Future Looks Like

through a Spine Oncology Lens." *Annals of Translational Medicine* 7(10): 224. https://doi.org/10.21037/atm.2019.04.69.

11. Hanley, Sharita. 2022. "What Is Surgical Oncology?" WebMD. https://www.webmd.com/cancer/what-is-surgical-oncology.

12. American Cancer Society. 2019. "How Surgery Is Used for Cancer." https://www.cancer.org/treatment/treatments-and-side-effects/treatment-types/surgery/how-surgery-is-used-for-cancer.html.

CHAPTER 10

1. American Society of Clinical Oncology. 2022. "What Is Chemotherapy?" Cancer.Net. https://www.cancer.net/navigating-cancer-care/how-cancer-treated/chemotherapy/what-chemotherapy.

2. American Cancer Society. 2019. "How Chemotherapy Drugs Work." https://www.cancer.org/treatment/treatments-and-side-effects/treatment-types/chemotherapy/how-chemotherapy-drugs-work.html.

3. American Cancer Society. 2020. "Chemotherapy Side Effects." https://www.cancer.org/treatment/treatments-and-side-effects/treatment-types/chemotherapy/chemotherapy-side-effects.html.

4. National Cancer Institute. n.d. "Side Effects of Cancer Treatment." https://www.cancer.gov/about-cancer/treatment/side-effects. Accessed Nov. 12, 2023.

CHAPTER 11

1. Chodos, Alan. 2001. "November 8, 1895: Roentgen's Discovery of X-Rays." American Physical Society. https://www.aps.org/publications/apsnews/200111/history.cfm.

2. The Nobel Prize. 2019. "Marie Curie." NobelPrize.org. https://www.nobelprize.org/prizes/physics/1903/marie-curie/facts/.

3. Wikipedia. 2018. "Marie Curie." https://en.wikipedia.org/wiki/Marie_Curie. Last modified Dec. 11, 2023.

4. Cho, Byungchul. 2018. "Intensity-Modulated Radiation Therapy: A Review with a Physics Perspective." *Radiation Oncology Journal* 36(1): 1–10. https://doi.org/10.3857/roj.2018.00122.

5. Taylor, A. 2004. "Intensity-Modulated Radiotherapy—What Is It?" *Cancer Imaging* 4(2): 68–73. https://doi.org/10.1102/1470-7330.2004.0003.

6. Jalil ur Rehman, Zahra, Nisar Ahmad, Muhammad Khalid, H. M. Noor ul Huda Khan Asghar, Zaheer Abbas Gilani, Irfan Ullah, Gulfam Nasar, et al. 2018. "Intensity Modulated Radiation Therapy: A Review of Current Practice and Future Outlooks." *Journal of Radiation Research and Applied Sciences* 11(4): 361–67. https://doi.org/10.1016/j.jrras.2018.07.006.

7. Radiological Society of North America and American College of Radiology. 2023. "Intensity-Modulated Radiation Therapy (IMRT)." RadiologyInfo.org. https://www.radiologyinfo.org/en/info/imrt. Last modified May 1, 2023.

8. American Society of Clinical Oncology. 2022. "What Is Radiation Therapy?" Cancer.Net. https://www.cancer.net/navigating-cancer-care/how-cancer-treated/radiation-therapy/what-radiation-therapy.

9. Wikipedia. 2023. "Tomotherapy." https://en.wikipedia.org/wiki/Tomotherapy. Last modified Oct. 10, 2023.

10. Fenwick, John D., Wolfgang A. Tomé, Emilie T. Soisson, Minesh P. Mehta, and Thomas R. Mackie. 2006. "Tomotherapy and Other Innovative IMRT Delivery Systems." *Seminars in Radiation Oncology* 16(4): 199–208. https://doi.org/10.1016/j.semradonc.2006.04.002.

11. Beavis, Andrew W. 2004. "Is Tomotherapy the Future of IMRT?" *British Journal of Radiology* 77(916): 285–95. https://doi.org/10.1259/bjr/22666727.

12. American Society of Clinical Oncology. 2022. "Proton Therapy." Cancer.Net. https://www.cancer.net/navigating-cancer-care/how-cancer-treated/radiation-therapy/proton-therapy.

13. RadiologyInfo.org. 2023. "Stereotactic Radiosurgery (SRS) and Stereotactic Body Radiotherapy (SBRT)." https://www.radiologyinfo.org/en/info/stereotactic. Last modified May 1, 2023.

14. Kurup, Gopalakrishna. 2010. "CyberKnife: A New Paradigm in Radiotherapy." *Journal of Medical Physics* 35(2): 63. https://doi.org/10.4103/0971-6203.62194.

15. RadiologyInfo.org. 2023. "Gamma Knife." https://www.radiologyinfo.org/en/info/gamma_knife. Last modified Aug. 30, 2023.

16. Skowronek, Janusz. 2017. "Current Status of Brachytherapy in Cancer Treatment—Short Overview." *Journal of Contemporary Brachytherapy* 9(6): 581–89. https://doi.org/10.5114/jcb.2017.72607.

17. National Cancer Institute. 2022. "Radiation Therapy Side Effects." https://www.cancer.gov/about-cancer/treatment/types/radiation-therapy/side-effects.

CHAPTER 12

1. At the Forefront. 1997. "Charles B. Huggins, MD, 1901–1997." UChicago Medicine. https://www.uchicagomedicine.org/forefront/news/charles-b--huggins-md-1901-1997.

2. The Nobel Prize. n.d. "Charles B. Huggins." https://www.nobelprize.org/prizes/medicine/1966/huggins/facts/. Accessed Nov. 12, 2023.

3. Nelson, William G. 2016. "Commentary on Huggins and Hodges: 'Studies on Prostatic Cancer.'" *Cancer Research* 76(2): 186–87. https://doi.org/10.1158/0008-5472.can-15-3172.

4. Huggins, C., and C. V. Hodges. 1972. "Studies on Prostatic Cancer: I. The Effect of Castration, of Estrogen and of Androgen Injection on Serum Phosphatases in Metastatic Carcinoma of the Prostate." *CA: A Cancer Journal for Clinicians* 22(4): 232–40. https://doi.org/10.3322/canjclin.22.4.232.

5. National Cancer Institute. 2021. "Hormonal Therapy for Prostate Cancer." https://www.cancer.gov/types/prostate/prostate-hormone-therapy-fact-sheet.

6. Garje Rohan, Adithya Chennamadhavuni, Sarah L. Mott, Isaac Matthew Chambers, Paul Gellhaus, Yousef Zakharia, and James A. Brown. 2020. "Utilization and Outcomes of Surgical Castration in Comparison to Medical Castration in Metastatic Prostate Cancer." *Clinical Genitourinary Cancer* 18(2): e157–66. https://doi.org/10.1016/j.clgc.2019.09.020.

7. Crawford, E. David, Axel Heidenreich, Nathan Lawrentschuk, Bertrand Tombal, Antonio C. L. Pompeo, Arturo Mendoza-Valdes, Kurt Miller, Frans M. J. Debruyne, and Laurence Klotz. 2018. "Androgen-Targeted Therapy in Men with Prostate Cancer: Evolving Practice and Future Considerations." *Prostate Cancer and Prostatic Diseases* 22(1): 24–38. https://doi.org/10.1038/s41391-018-0079-0.

8. Hussain, Maha, Catherine M. Tangen, Donna L. Berry, Celestia S. Higano, E. David Crawford, Glenn Liu, George Wilding, et al. 2013. "Intermittent versus Continuous Androgen Deprivation in Prostate Cancer." *New England Journal of Medicine* 368(14): 1314–25. https://doi.org/10.1056/nejmoa1212299.

9. Shute, Nancy. 2013. "The Last Word on Hormone Therapy from the Women's Health Initiative." NPR.org. https://www.npr.org/sections/health-shots/2013/10/04/229171477/the-last-word-on-hormone-therapy-from-the-womens-health-initiative.

10. University of Oxford; Oxford Population Health. n.d. "The Million Women Study." http://www.millionwomenstudy.org/introduction/. Accessed Nov. 12, 2023.

11. Writing Group for the Women's Health Initiative Investigators. 2002. "Risks and Benefits of Estrogen plus Progestin in Healthy Postmenopausal Women: Principal Results from the Women's Health Initiative Randomized Controlled Trial." *JAMA* 288 (3): 321–33. https://doi.org/10.1001/jama.288.3.321.

12. Gilmore, Ron. 2014. "'Father of Tamoxifen.'" MD Anderson Cancer Center. https://www.mdanderson.org/publications/promise/father-of-tamoxifen-craig-jordan.h36-1589046.html.

13. Khetrapal, Afsaneh. 2021. "Tamoxifen Discovery." News-Medical.net. https://www.news-medical.net/health/Tamoxifen-Discovery.aspx.

14. Cosman, Felicia, and Robert Lindsay. 2007. "Selective Estrogen Receptor Modulator." ScienceDirect. https://www.sciencedirect.com/topics/medicine-and-dentistry/selective-estrogen-receptor-modulator.

15. American Cancer Society. 2021. "Tamoxifen and Raloxifene for Lowering Breast Cancer Risk." Cancer.org. https://www.cancer.org/cancer/breast-cancer/risk-and-prevention/tamoxifen-and-raloxifene-for-breast-cancer-prevention.html.

16. American Cancer Society. 2021. "Aromatase Inhibitors for Lowering Breast Cancer Risk." https://www.cancer.org/cancer/breast-cancer/risk-and-prevention/aromatase-inhibitors-for-lowering-breast-cancer-risk.html.

17. Gnant, Michael, Florian Fitzal, Gabriel Rinnerthaler, Guenther G. Steger, Sigrun Greil-Ressler, Marija Balic, Dietmar Heck, et al. 2021. "Duration of Adjuvant Aromatase-Inhibitor Therapy in Postmenopausal Breast Cancer." *New England Journal of Medicine* 385(5): 395–405. https://doi.org/10.1056/nejmoa2104162.

CHAPTER 13

1. American Society of Clinical Oncology. 2022. "What Is Targeted Therapy?" Cancer.Net. https://www.cancer.net/navigating-cancer-care/how-cancer-treated/personalized-and-targeted-therapies/what-targeted-therapy.

2. Coiffier, Bertrand, Eric Lepage, Josette Brière, Raoul Herbrecht, Hervé Tilly, Reda Bouabdallah, Pierre Morel, et al. 2002. "CHOP Chemotherapy plus Rituximab Compared with CHOP Alone in Elderly Patients with Diffuse Large-B-Cell Lymphoma." *New England Journal of Medicine* 346(4): 235–42. https://doi.org/10.1056/nejmoa011795.

3. Biba, Erin. n.d. "The HER2 Journey." Genentech. https://www.gene.com/stories/her2/. Accessed Nov. 12, 2023.

4. UChicago News. 2013. "Janet Rowley, Cancer Genetics Pioneer, 1925–2013." University of Chicago News. https://news.uchicago.edu/story/janet-rowley-cancer-genetics-pioneer-1925-2013.

5. Rowley, Janet D. 1973. "A New Consistent Chromosomal Abnormality in Chronic Myelogenous Leukaemia Identified by Quinacrine Fluorescence and Giemsa Staining." *Nature* 243(5405): 290–93. https://doi.org/10.1038/243290a0.

6. Golomb, Harvey M., and Janet D. Rowley. 1981. "Significance of Cytogenetic Abnormalities in Acute Leukemias." *Human Pathology* 12(6): 515–22. https://doi.org/10.1016/s0046-8177(81)80065-2.

7. Le Beau, Michelle M., Carol A. Westbrook, Manuel O. Diaz, Janet D. Rowley, and Moshe Oren. 1985. "Translocation of the p53 Gene in T(15;17) in Acute Promyelocytic Leukaemia." *Nature* 316(6031): 826–28. https://doi.org/10.1038/316826a0.

8. Nowell, Peter C. 2007. "Discovery of the Philadelphia Chromosome: A Personal Perspective." *Journal of Clinical Investigation* 117(8): 2033–35. https://doi.org/10.1172/jci31771.

9. National Cancer Institute. 2018. "Angiogenesis Inhibitors." https://www
.cancer.gov/about-cancer/treatment/types/immunotherapy/angiogenesis
-inhibitors-fact-sheet.

10. Shepherd, Frances A., José Rodrigues Pereira, Tudor Ciuleanu, Eng Huat
Tan, Vera Hirsh, Sumitra Thongprasert, Daniel Campos, et al. 2005.
"Erlotinib in Previously Treated Non–Small-Cell Lung Cancer." *New
England Journal of Medicine* 353(2): 123–32. https://doi.org/10.1056
/nejmoa050753.

CHAPTER 14

1. Dahlén, Eva, Niina Veitonmäki, and Per Norlén. 2018. "Bispecific
Antibodies in Cancer Immunotherapy." *Therapeutic Advances in
Vaccines and Immunotherapy* 6(1): 3–17. https://doi.org/10.1177/25151355
18763280.

2. Weiner, Louis M., Madhav V. Dhodapkar, and Soldano Ferrone. 2009.
"Monoclonal Antibodies for Cancer Immunotherapy." *The Lancet*
373(9668): 1033–40. https://doi.org/10.1016/s0140-6736(09)60251-8.

3. Cancer Research Institute. 2015. "Checkpoint Inhibitors: Taking the
Brakes off the Immune System." YouTube. https://www.youtube.com
/watch?v=v9NBUeU3PG0.

4. Langer, Julia. 2021. "How Immunotherapy Is like an Old Western Movie."
The Skin Cancer Foundation. https://www.skincancer.org/blog/how
-immunotherapy-is-like-an-old-western-movie/.

5. Kantoff, Philip W., Celestia S. Higano, Neal D. Shore, E. Roy Berger,
Eric J. Small, David F. Penson, Charles H. Redfern, et al. 2010. "Sipuleucel-T
Immunotherapy for Castration-Resistant Prostate Cancer." *New England
Journal of Medicine* 363(5): 411–22. https://doi.org/10.1056/nejmoa1001294.

6. Ferrucci, Pier Francesco, Laura Pala, Fabio Conforti, and Emilia Cocoroc-
chio. 2021. "Talimogene Laherparepvec (T-VEC): An Intralesional Cancer
Immunotherapy for Advanced Melanoma." *Cancers* 13(6): 1383. https://doi
.org/10.3390/cancers13061383.

7. National Cancer Institute. 2018. "Using Oncolytic Viruses to Treat Cancer."
https://www.cancer.gov/news-events/cancer-currents-blog/2018/oncolytic
-viruses-to-treat-cancer.

8. Singhal, Seema, Jayesh Mehta, Raman Desikan, Dan Ayers, Paula Roberson, Paul Eddlemon, Nikhil Munshi, et al. 1999. "Antitumor Activity of Thalidomide in Refractory Multiple Myeloma." *New England Journal of Medicine* 341(21): 1565–71. https://doi.org/10.1056/nejm199911183412102.

9. Sheikhbahaei, Sara, Charles Marcus, Mohammad Salehi Sadaghiani, Steven P. Rowe, Martin G. Pomper, and Lilja B. Solnes. 2022. "Imaging of Cancer Immunotherapy: Response Assessment Methods, Atypical Response Patterns, and Immune-Related Adverse Events, from the *AJR* Special Series on Imaging of Inflammation." *American Journal of Roentgenology* 218(6): 940–52. https://doi.org/10.2214/ajr.21.26538.

10. Somarouthu, Bhanusupriya, Susanna I. Lee, Trinity Urban, Cheryl A. Sadow, Gordon J. Harris, and Avinash Kambadakone. 2018. "Immune-Related Tumour Response Assessment Criteria: A Comprehensive Review." *British Journal of Radiology* 91(1084): 20170457. https://doi.org/10.1259/bjr.20170457.

11. Ma, Yiming, Qiwei Wang, Qian Dong, Lei Zhan, and Jingdong Zhang. 2019. "How to Differentiate Pseudoprogression from True Progression in Cancer Patients Treated with Immunotherapy." *American Journal of Cancer Research* 9(8): 1546–53. https://www.ncbi.nlm.nih.gov/pmc/articles/PMC6726978/.

CHAPTER 15

1. National Marrow Donor Program. 2018. "What Is a Bone Marrow Transplant?" https://bethematch.org/patients-and-families/about-transplant/what-is-a-bone-marrow-transplant-/.

2. American Society of Clinical Oncology. 2020. "What Is a Bone Marrow Transplant (Stem Cell Transplant)?" Cancer.Net. https://www.cancer.net/navigating-cancer-care/how-cancer-treated/bone-marrowstem-cell-transplantation/what-bone-marrow-transplant-stem-cell-transplant.

3. National Marrow Donor Program. n.d. "HLA Basics." https://bethematch.org/transplant-basics/how-blood-stem-cell-transplants-work/hla-basics/. Accessed Nov. 12, 2023.

4. American Cancer Society. 2020. "Stem Cell or Bone Marrow Transplant Side Effects." Cancer.org. https://www.cancer.org/treatment/treatments-and-side-effects/treatment-types/stem-cell-transplant/transplant-side-effects.html.

5. Senzolo, M., G. Germani, E. Cholongitas, P. Burra, and A. K. Burroughs. 2007. "Veno Occlusive Disease: Update on Clinical Management." *World Journal of Gastroenterology* 13(29): 3918–24. https://doi.org/10.3748/wjg.v13.i29.3918.

6. Justiz Vaillant, Angel A., and Oranus Mohammadi. 2020. "Graft versus Host Disease." PubMed. Treasure Island, FL: StatPearls Publishing. Last modified Oct. 2021. https://www.ncbi.nlm.nih.gov/books/NBK538235/.

7. National Marrow Donor Program. n.d. "Graft-versus-Host Disease Basics." https://bethematch.org/patients-and-families/life-after-transplant/physical-health-and-recovery/graft-versus-host-disease-basics/. Accessed Nov. 12, 2023.

8. National Cancer Institute. n.d. "CAR T-Cell Therapy." In *NCI Dictionary of Cancer Terms*. https://www.cancer.gov/publications/dictionaries/cancer-terms/def/car-t-cell-therapy. Accessed Nov. 12, 2023.

9. The Emily Whitehead Foundation. n.d. "Our Journey." https://emilywhiteheadfoundation.org/our-journey/. Accessed Nov. 12, 2023.

10. Neff Newitt, Valerie. 2022. "The Incredible Story of Emily Whitehead & CAR T-Cell Therapy." *Oncology Times* 44(6): 1, 19–21. https://doi.org/10.1097/01.cot.0000824668.24475.b0.

11. Filley, Anna C., Mario Henriquez, and Mahua Dey. 2018. "CART Immunotherapy: Development, Success, and Translation to Malignant Gliomas and Other Solid Tumors." *Frontiers in Oncology* 8(8): 453. https://doi.org/10.3389/fonc.2018.00453.

12. Maude, Shannon L., Theodore W. Laetsch, Jochen Buechner, Susana Rives, Michael Boyer, Henrique Bittencourt, Peter Bader, et al. 2018. "Tisagenlecleucel in Children and Young Adults with B-Cell Lymphoblastic Leukemia." *New England Journal of Medicine* 378(5): 439–48. https://doi.org/10.1056/nejmoa1709866.

13. Neelapu, Sattva S., Frederick L. Locke, Nancy L. Bartlett, Lazaros J. Lekakis, David B. Miklos, Caron A. Jacobson, Ira Braunschweig, et al. 2017. "Axicabtagene Ciloleucel CAR T-Cell Therapy in Refractory Large B-Cell Lymphoma." *New England Journal of Medicine* 377(26): 2531–44. https://doi.org/10.1056/nejmoa1707447.

14. Schuster, Stephen J., Michael R. Bishop, Constantine S. Tam, Edmund K. Waller, Peter Borchmann, Joseph P. McGuirk, Ulrich Jäger, et al. 2019. "Tisagenlecleucel in Adult Relapsed or Refractory Diffuse Large B-Cell Lymphoma." *New England Journal of Medicine* 380(1): 45–56. https://doi.org/10.1056/nejmoa1804980.

15. Kamdar, Manali, Scott R. Solomon, Jon Arnason, Patrick B. Johnston, Bertram Glass, Veronika Bachanova, Sami Ibrahimi, et al. 2022. "Lisocabtagene Maraleucel versus Standard of Care with Salvage Chemotherapy Followed by Autologous Stem Cell Transplantation as Second-Line Treatment in Patients with Relapsed or Refractory Large B-Cell Lymphoma (TRANSFORM): Results from an Interim Analysis of an Open-Label, Randomised, Phase 3 Trial." *Lancet* 399(10343): 2294–308. https://doi.org/10.1016/S0140-6736(22)00662-6.

16. National Cancer Institute staff. 2022. "Should CAR T Cells Be Used Earlier in People with Non-Hodgkin Lymphoma?" *Cancer Currents* (blog). https://www.cancer.gov/news-events/cancer-currents-blog/2022/nhl-car-t-cells-belinda-transform-zuma7.

17. Bishop, Michael R., Michael Dickinson, Duncan Purtill, Pere Barba, Armando Santoro, Nada Hamad, Koji Kato, et al. 2021. "Second-Line Tisagenlecleucel or Standard Care in Aggressive B-Cell Lymphoma." *New England Journal of Medicine* 386(December): 629–39. https://doi.org/10.1056/nejmoa2116596.

18. Locke, Frederick L., David B. Miklos, Caron A. Jacobson, Miguel-Angel Perales, Marie-José Kersten, Olalekan O. Oluwole, Armin Ghobadi, et al. 2022. "Axicabtagene Ciloleucel as Second-Line Therapy for Large B-Cell Lymphoma." *New England Journal of Medicine* 386(February): 640–54. https://doi.org/10.1056/nejmoa2116133.

19. Frey, Noelle, and David Porter. 2019. "Cytokine Release Syndrome with Chimeric Antigen Receptor T Cell Therapy." *Biology of Blood and Marrow Transplantation* 25(4): e123–27. https://doi.org/10.1016/j.bbmt.2018.12.756.

20. Siegler, Elizabeth L., and Saad S. Kenderian. 2020. "Neurotoxicity and Cytokine Release Syndrome after Chimeric Antigen Receptor T Cell Therapy: Insights into Mechanisms and Novel Therapies." *Frontiers in Immunology* 11(August): 1973. https://doi.org/10.3389/fimmu.2020.01973.

21. Hu, Yongxian, Jingjing Li, Fang Ni, Zhongli Yang, Xiaohua Gui, Zhiwei Bao, Houli Zhao, et al. 2022. "CAR-T Cell Therapy-Related Cytokine Release Syndrome and Therapeutic Response Is Modulated by the Gut Microbiome in Hematologic Malignancies." *Nature Communications* 13(1): 5313. https://doi.org/10.1038/s41467-022-32960-3.

CHAPTER 16

1. National Cancer Institute. 2023. "Complementary and Alternative Medicine." https://www.cancer.gov/about-cancer/treatment/cam.

2. Benzinga. 2023. "Complementary and Alternative Medicine Market Expected to Reach USD 362.97 Bn by 2029 at a Growth Rate of 17.9 Percent." EIN News, March 13, 2023. https://www.einnews.com/pr_news/621867748/complementary-and-alternative-medicine-market-expected-to-reach-usd-362-97-bn-by-2029-at-a-growth-rate-of-17-9-percent.

3. American Cancer Society. n.d. "Dietary Supplements." https://www.cancer.org/treatment/treatments-and-side-effects/treatment-types/complementary-and-integrative-medicine/dietary-supplements.html. Accessed Nov. 12, 2023.

4. Cancer Research UK. 2022. "Vitamins, Diet Supplements, and Cancer." https://www.cancerresearchuk.org/about-cancer/treatment/complementary-alternative-therapies/individual-therapies/vitamins-diet-supplements.

5. National Cancer Institute. Cancer Trends Progress Report. 2023. "Red Meat and Processed Meat Consumption." https://progressreport.cancer.gov/prevention/red_meat. Accessed Nov. 12, 2023.

6. Cancer Research UK. 2022. "Wholegrains, Fibre, and Cancer Risk." https://www.cancerresearchuk.org/about-cancer/causes-of-cancer/diet-and-cancer/wholegrains-fibre-and-cancer-risk.

7. Centers for Disease Control and Prevention. 2023. "Alcohol and Cancer." https://www.cdc.gov/cancer/alcohol/index.htm.

8. Cancer Council. n.d. "Does Sugar Cause Cancer?" Cancer.org.au. https://www.cancer.org.au/iheard/does-sugar-cause-cancer. Accessed Nov. 12, 2023.

9.   Cancer Research UK. 2023. "Sugar and Cancer—What You Need to Know." https://news.cancerresearchuk.org/2020/10/20/sugar-and-cancer-what -you-need-to-know/. Accessed Nov. 12, 2023.

10. National Cancer Institute. "Artificial Sweeteners and Cancer." n.d. https://www.cancer.gov/about-cancer/causes-prevention/risk/diet /artificial-sweeteners-fact-sheet#r1. Accessed Jan. 29, 2024.

11. Filippini, Tommaso, Marcella Malavolyi, Francesca Borrelli, Angelo A. Izzo, Susan J. Fairweather-Tait, Markus Horneber, and Marco Vinceti. 2020. "Green Tea (Camellia Sinensis) for the Prevention of Cancer." *Cochrane Database of Systematic Reviews* 3(3): CD005004. https://doi.org/10 .1002/14651858.CD005004.pub3.

12. Cancer Research UK. n.d. "Green Tea (Chinese Tea)." https://www.can cerresearchuk.org/about-cancer/treatment/complementary-alternative -therapies/individual-therapies/green-tea. Accessed Nov. 12, 2023.

13. National Cancer Institute. 2022. "Eating Hints: Before, during, and after Cancer Treatment." https://www.cancer.gov/publications/patient-educa tion/eatinghints.pdf.

14. Cassileth, Barrie R. 2010. "Saw Palmetto." Cancer Network. https://www .cancernetwork.com/view/saw-palmetto.

15. Baudry, Julia, Karen E. Assmann, Mathilde Touvier, Benjamin Alles, Louise Seconda, Paule Latino-Martel, Khaled Ezzedine, et al. 2018. "Association of Frequency of Organic Food Consumption with Cancer: Findings from the Nutrient-Sante Prospective Cohort Study." *JAMA Internal Medicine* 178(12): 1597–606. https://doi.org/10.1001/jamainternmed.2018.4357.

16. American Cancer Society. 2022. "Marijuana and Cancer." https://www .cancer.org/treatment/treatments-and-side-effects/treatment-types /complementary-and-integrative-medicine/marijuana-and-cancer.html.

17. National Cancer Institute. 2023. "Cannabis and Cannabinoids (PDQ®)– Patient Version." https://www.cancer.gov/about-cancer/treatment/cam /patient/cannabis-pdq. Accessed Nov. 12, 2023.

18. Mehta, Ria, Kirti Sharma, Louis Potters, A. Gabriella Wernicke, and Bhupesh Parashar. 2019. "Evidence for the Role of Mindfulness in Cancer: Benefits and Techniques." *Cureus* 11(5): e4629–41. https://doi.org/10.7759/cureus.4629.

19. National Cancer Institute. 2023. "Acupuncture (PDQ®)–Patient Version." https://www.cancer.gov/about-cancer/treatment/cam/patient/acupuncture -pdq. Accessed Nov. 12, 2023.

20. National Center for Complementary and Integrative Health. 2022. "Acupuncture: What You Need to Know." https://www.nccih.nih.gov /health/acupuncture-what-you-need-to-know.

21. American Cancer Society. 2022. "Physical Activity and the Person with Cancer." https://www.cancer.org/treatment/survivorship-during-and -after-treatment/be-healthy-after-treatment/physical-activity-and-the -cancer-patient.html.

22. Monika Stanczyk, Malgorzata. 2011. "Music Therapy in Supportive Cancer Care." *Reports of Practical Oncology and Radiotherapy* 16(5): 170–72. https://doi.org/10.1016/j.rpor.2011.04.005.

23. American Cancer Society. 2023. "Pets, Support, and Service Animals for People with Cancer." https://www.cancer.org/treatment/survivorship -during-and-after-treatment/coping/support-service-animals.html. Accessed Nov. 12, 2023.

24. Li, Kailimi, Linman Weng, and Xueqiang Wang. 2021. "The State of Music Therapy Studies in the Past 20 Years: A Bibliometric Analysis." *Frontiers in Psychology* 12:697726. https://doi.org/10.3389/fpsyg.2021 .697726.

25. Bradt, Joke, Cheryl Dileo, Katherine Myers-Coffman, and Jacelyn Biondo. 2021. "Music Interventions for Improving Psychological and Physical Outcomes in People with Cancer." *Cochrane Database of Systematic Reviews* 10(10): CD006911. https://doi.org/10.1002/14651858.CD006911 .pub4.

26. Hansten, Philip D. 2018. "The Underrated Risks of Tamoxifen Drug Interactions." *European Journal of Drug Metabolis and Pharmacokinetics* 43(5): 495–508. https://doi.org/10.1007/s13318-018-0475-9.

CHAPTER 17

1. National Institute on Aging. 2021. "What Are Palliative Care and Hospice Care?" https://www.nia.nih.gov/health/what-are-palliative-care-and -hospice-care.

2. National Cancer Institute. 2021. "Palliative Care in Cancer." https://www
.cancer.gov/about-cancer/advanced-cancer/care-choices/palliative-care-fact
-sheet.

3. Sullivan, Donald R., Benjamin Chan, Jodi A. Lapidus, Linda Ganzini, Lissi
Hansen, Patricia A. Carney, Erik K. Fromme, et al. 2019. "Association of
Early Palliative Care Use with Survival and Place of Death among Patients
with Advanced Lung Cancer Receiving Care in the Veterans Health Administration." *JAMA Oncology* 5(12): 1702–9. https://doi.org/10.1001/jama
oncol.2019.3105.

4. Temel, Jennifer S., Joseph A. Greer, Alona Muzikansky, Emily R. Galla-
gher, Sonal Admane, Vicki A. Jackson, Constance M. Dahlin, et al. 2010.
"Early Palliative Care for Patients with Metastatic Non–Small-Cell Lung
Cancer." *New England Journal of Medicine* 363(8): 733–42. https://doi.org/10
.1056/NEJMoa1000678.

CHAPTER 18

1. Meyerhardt, Jeffrey A., Pamela B. Mangu, Patrick J. Flynn, Larissa
Korde, Charles L. Loprinzi, Bruce D. Minsky, Nicholas J. Petrelli, et al.
2013. "Follow-Up Care, Surveillance Protocol, and Secondary Prevention
Measures for Survivors of Colorectal Cancer: American Society of Clinical
Oncology Clinical Practice Guideline Endorsement." *Journal of Clinical
Oncology* 31(35). https://doi.org/10.1200/JCO.2013.50.7442.

CHAPTER 21

1. National Cancer Institute. n.d. "Survivorship." https://www.cancer.gov
/publications/dictionaries/cancer-terms/def/survivorship. Accessed
Nov. 12, 2023.

2. American Society of Clinical Oncology. 2021. "What Is Cancer Survivorship?" Cancer.Net. https://www.cancer.net/survivorship/what-cancer
-survivorship.

3. Denlinger, Crystal S., Robert W. Carlson, Madhuri Are, K. Scott Baker,
Elizabeth Davis, Stephen B. Edge, Debra L. Friedman, et al. 2015. "Survi-
vorship: Introduction and Definition." *Journal of the National Comprehensive
Cancer Network* 12(1): 35–45. doi: 10.6004/jnccn.2014.0005.

4. Siegel, Rebecca L., Kimberkly D. Miller, Hannah E. Fuchs, Ahmedin Jemal. 2022. "Cancer Statistics." *CA: A Cancer Journal for Clinicians* 72(1): 7–33. https://doi.org/10.3322/caac.21708.

5. National Cancer Institute. 2022. "Statistics and Graphs." https://cancer control.cancer.gov/ocs/statistics#stats.

6. American Society of Clinical Oncology. 2014. "ASCO Guideline Adaptation of a Pan-Canadian Practice Guideline: Screening, Assessment and Care of Psychosocial Distress (Depression, Anxiety) in Adults with Cancer." https://old-prod.asco.org/sites/new-www.asco.org/files/content-files/practice-and-guidelines/documents/depression-anxiety-summary-of-recs-table.pdf.

7. American Society of Clinical Oncology. n.d. "ASCO Cancer Treatment and Survivorship Care Plans." Cancer.Net. https://www.cancer.net/survivorship/follow-care-after-cancer-treatment/asco-cancer-treatment-and-survivorship-care-plans. Accessed Nov. 12, 2023.

8. US Department of Labor. n.d. "Family and Medical Leave Act." https://www.dol.gov/agencies/whd/fmla. Accessed Nov. 12, 2023.

9. National Network Information, Guidance, and Training on the Americans with Disabilities Act. 2023. "What Is the Americans with Disabilities Act (ADA)?" https://adata.org/learn-about-ada. Accessed Nov. 12, 2023.

10. US Department of Labor. n.d. "Americans with Disabilities Act." https://www.dol.gov/general/topic/disability/ada. Accessed Nov. 12, 2023.

11. National Cancer Institute. 2022. "Financial Toxicity and Cancer Treatment (PDQ®)–Health Professional Version." https://www.cancer.gov/about-cancer/managing-care/track-care-costs/financial-toxicity-hp-pdq.

CHAPTER 22

1. Health Resources and Services Administration. n.d. "Billing for Telehealth." Telehealth.HHS.gov. https://telehealth.hhs.gov/providers/billing-and-reimbursement. Accessed Nov. 12, 2023.

2. Health Resources and Services Administration. n.d. "What Is Telehealth?" Telehealth.HHS.gov. https://telehealth.hhs.gov/patients/understanding-telehealth. Accessed Nov. 12, 2023.

3. US Food and Drug Administration. 2023. "Real-World Evidence." https://www.fda.gov/science-research/science-and-research-special-topics/real-world-evidence. Accessed Nov. 12, 2023.

4. US Food and Drug Administration. 2018. "Surrogate Endpoint Resources for Drug and Biologic Development." https://www.fda.gov/drugs/development-resources/surrogate-endpoint-resources-drug-and-biologic-development.

5. US Food and Drug Administration. 2020. "21st Century Cures Act." https://www.fda.gov/regulatory-information/selected-amendments-fdc-act/21st-century-cures-act.

6. US Food and Drug Administration. 2022. "Focus Area: Patient-Reported Outcomes and Other Clinical Outcome Assessments." https://www.fda.gov/science-research/focus-areas-regulatory-science-report/focus-area-patient-reported-outcomes-and-other-clinical-outcome-assessments.

7. Basch, Ethan, Allison M. Deal, Amylou C. Dueck, Howard I. Scher, Mark G. Kris, Clifford Hudis, and Deborah Schrag. 2017. "Overall Survival Results of a Trial Assessing Patient-Reported Outcomes for Symptom Monitoring during Routine Cancer Treatment." *JAMA* 318(2): 197–98. https://doi.org/10.1001/jama.2017.7156.

8. US Food and Drug Administration. 2023. "Accelerated Approval Program." https://www.fda.gov/drugs/nda-and-bla-approvals/accelerated-approval-program. Accessed Nov. 12, 2023.

9. Senate Democratic Caucus. 2022. "Summary: The Inflation Reduction Act of 2022." https://www.democrats.senate.gov/imo/media/doc/inflation_reduction_act_one_page_summary.pdf.

10. National Human Genome Research Institute. 2023. "The Human Genome Project." https://www.genome.gov/human-genome-project. Accessed Nov. 12, 2023.

11. Behjati, Sam, and Patrick S. Tarpey. 2013. "What Is Next Generation Sequencing?" *Archives of Disease in Childhood: Education and Practice Edition* 98(6): 236–38. https://doi.org/10.1136/archdischild-2013-304340.

Index

pre-surgery questions and, 108;
real-world data from, 292;
screening and, 24; second
opinions and, 82–83; telehealth
and, 289
integrative oncology, 213–14
intensity-modulated radiation
therapy (IMRT), 125
interferons, 166, 167
interleukin 2, 167
interleukins, 166
internal radiation therapy, 129
International Agency for Research
on Cancer (IARC), 204
International Congress on
Malignant Lymphoma, 2
interventional radiologists, 49–50
intraoperative radiation, 129
intrathecal therapy, 117
intravenous chemotherapy delivery,
115–16; dosage calculations in,
118; verifying delivery of, 119
intravenous fluids (IV fluids), 225–26

Jordan, V. Craig, 144, 145
June, Carl, 194

Kahneman, Daniel, 106
keloids, 125
ketoconazole, 141
ketogenic diet, 205–6
ketosis, 205
kidney cancer, 41, 43, 74, 214, 216,
236; interleukins and, 167
K-RAS gene, 300

laboratory studies: for monitoring
for recurrence, 236; staging
and, 68

LAG-3 checkpoint, 163
language barriers, 265, 269
laparoscopic surgery, 104
large B-cell lymphoma, 149, 279;
diffuse, 91–92
large-cell lymphoma, 276–77
larotrectinib (Vitrakvi), 303
laser surgery, 105
Leksell, Lars, 128
letrozole (Femara), 146
leukapheresis, 190
leukemia, 13, 172, 173, 265–67;
acute lymphoblastic, 194; acute
myeloid, 66, 162, 245; acute
promyelocytic, 154; chromosome
translocations and, 298; chronic
lymphocytic, 47, 65–66, 205;
chronic myelogenous, 153–54,
298; chronic myeloid, 88–89,
152, 181
leuprolide (Lupron), 140
lifestyle: cancer risks and, 13; obesity
and, 15
linear accelerator (LINAC), 124
liquid biopsy, 51, 301
liquid tumors, 68
liver cancer, hepatitis B virus and, 166
Livestrong Foundation, 67
local recurrence, 238
long-term follow-up care, 279–81
lorazepam (Ativan), 227–28
low-dose CT scans, 34
lung cancer, 8–9, 222, 228, 238–40,
273–74; non-small cell, 158;
screening for, 22, 33–35; signs
and symptoms, 41; staging, 68,
75; targeted therapies and, 157,
158–59; tobacco and, 14–15;
treatment of, 75, 99

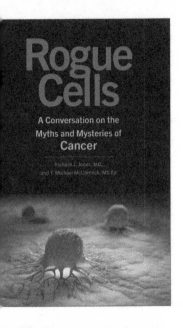
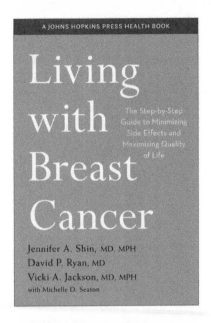
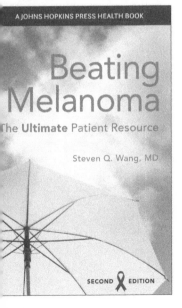
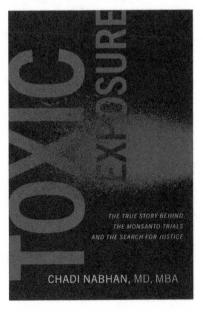